CAMBRIDGE LIBRARY COLLECTION

Books of enduring scholarly value

History of Medicine

It is sobering to realise that as recently as the year in which On the Origin of Species was published, learned opinion was that diseases such as typhus and cholera were spread by a 'miasma', and suggestions that doctors should wash their hands before examining patients were greeted with mockery by the profession. The Cambridge Library Collection reissues milestone publications in the history of Western medicine as well as studies of other medical traditions. Its coverage ranges from Galen on anatomical procedures to Florence Nightingale's common-sense advice to nurses, and includes early research into genetics and mental health, colonial reports on tropical diseases, documents on public health and military medicine, and publications on spa culture and medicinal plants.

A Memoir of John Conolly

John Conolly (1794–1866) was a physician and alienist (psychiatrist) who worked with the mentally ill at the Hanwell County Asylum in Middlesex, where he introduced the principle of non-restraint. This action was at first controversial and met with strong opposition, but it served to further the cause of humane treatment, securing Conolly's reputation. Published in 1869, this biography was the last major work of Sir James Clark (1788–1870), a supporter of Conolly's enlightened methods. Clark himself had enjoyed a distinguished medical career, becoming a trusted physician and friend to Queen Victoria. Also reissued in this series are his *Medical Notes on Climate, Diseases, Hospitals, and Medical Schools in France, Italy, and Switzerland* (1820), *The Influence of Climate in the Prevention and Cure of Chronic Diseases* (1829) and *A Treatise on Pulmonary Consumption* (1835).

T0383911

Cambridge University Press has long been a pioneer in the reissuing of out-of-print titles from its own backlist, producing digital reprints of books that are still sought after by scholars and students but could not be reprinted economically using traditional technology. The Cambridge Library Collection extends this activity to a wider range of books which are still of importance to researchers and professionals, either for the source material they contain, or as landmarks in the history of their academic discipline.

Drawing from the world-renowned collections in the Cambridge University Library and other partner libraries, and guided by the advice of experts in each subject area, Cambridge University Press is using state-of-the-art scanning machines in its own Printing House to capture the content of each book selected for inclusion. The files are processed to give a consistently clear, crisp image, and the books finished to the high quality standard for which the Press is recognised around the world. The latest print-on-demand technology ensures that the books will remain available indefinitely, and that orders for single or multiple copies can quickly be supplied.

The Cambridge Library Collection brings back to life books of enduring scholarly value (including out-of-copyright works originally issued by other publishers) across a wide range of disciplines in the humanities and social sciences and in science and technology.

A Memoir of
John Conolly

*Comprising a Sketch of the Treatment
of the Insane in Europe and America*

JAMES CLARK

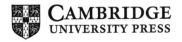

CAMBRIDGE
UNIVERSITY PRESS

CAMBRIDGE UNIVERSITY PRESS

Cambridge, New York, Melbourne, Madrid, Cape Town,
Singapore, São Paolo, Delhi, Mexico City

Published in the United States of America by Cambridge University Press, New York

www.cambridge.org
Information on this title: www.cambridge.org/9781108062497

© in this compilation Cambridge University Press 2013

This edition first published 1869
This digitally printed version 2013

ISBN 978-1-108-06249-7 Paperback

This book reproduces the text of the original edition. The content and language reflect
the beliefs, practices and terminology of their time, and have not been updated.

Cambridge University Press wishes to make clear that the book, unless originally published
by Cambridge, is not being republished by, in association or collaboration with, or
with the endorsement or approval of, the original publisher or its successors in title.

MEMOIR OF JOHN CONOLLY, M.D., D.C.L.

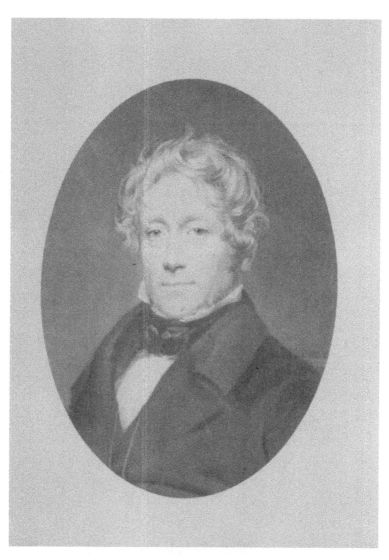

A MEMOIR

OF

JOHN CONOLLY, M.D., D.C.L.,

COMPRISING A SKETCH

OF THE

TREATMENT OF THE INSANE

IN

EUROPE AND AMERICA.

BY

SIR JAMES CLARK, Bart., K.C.B., M.D., F.R.S.,

PHYSICIAN IN ORDINARY TO THE QUEEN.

LONDON:

JOHN MURRAY, ALBEMARLE STREET.

1869.

LONDON: PRINTED BY W. CLOWES AND SONS, DUKE STREET, STAMFORD STREET,
AND CHARING CROSS.

TO THE

EARL OF SHAFTESBURY, K.G.,

CHAIRMAN OF THE COMMISSIONERS IN LUNACY.

My Lord,

In asking your Lordship to accept the dedication of the following Memoir, I have been actuated by several motives. You are pre-eminently the friend of the Insane; you were the friend of Dr. Conolly, and supported him in his arduous efforts to abolish mechanical restraints in the treatment of Lunacy; and, while I believe that the influence of your Lordship's name will have great effect in promoting the extension of the non-restraint system in those countries where it is not yet understood or appreciated, I am also afforded the opportunity of expressing my admiration of your Lordship's character, and the sincere esteem with which I have the honour to subscribe myself

Your Lordship's

Faithful Servant,

JAMES CLARK.

PREFACE.

WHEN the grave has closed over a man, the greater part of whose life has been devoted to works of benevolence, which have conferred a lasting benefit upon mankind, it is due to his memory that the public should be reminded of what he did, and of how he achieved his high objects.

Such a man was Dr. John Conolly, and it is the purpose of the following Memoir to give an account of his works—especially of that great work, which has ranked him among the benefactors of his race.

Dr. Conolly lived during a remarkable period in the medical history of insanity,—namely between the end of the last century, when Pinel first struck the shackles from the limbs of the lunatic, and the middle of the present century, when he himself put an end to the use of all forms of mechanical restraint in our asylums.

Dr. Conolly's work was one of years, and

was beset with difficulties, such as, but for the
possession of a rare combination of intellectual
and moral qualities, he never could have overcome.

In his endeavours to establish the system of
non-restraint in the treatment of the insane,
he no doubt received important assistance from
fellow-labourers in the same field,—and this he
always readily and cordially acknowledged. But
it was by his own energetic and persevering
labours in Hanwell Asylum, aided by his eloquent, powerful, and unremitting advocacy of
the cause, that he succeeded in placing non-
restraint on the firm and enduring basis which
it now occupies.

Although his chief object, perhaps, was the
care of the pauper lunatic, he lost sight of
nothing which could contribute to the well-
being and proper treatment of all classes of
the insane. His attention, for instance, was
long directed to the neglected condition of the
idiotic and imbecile; and the success of his
efforts in their behalf is disclosed in the following pages. Nor were his interest and sympathy confined to the unsound of mind, they
extended to every measure calculated to pro-

mote social progress, and to improve the position of the helpless classes generally.

In collecting materials for this Memoir, I have had the valuable assistance of Dr. Conolly's family, and of his sons-in-law Dr. Harrington Tuke and Dr. Maudsley. I am especially indebted for important information to an obituary notice written by Dr. Maudsley. My thanks are also due, in a particular manner, to Dr. Conolly's esteemed friend Monsieur Battel, for the use of many interesting letters; and I have to acknowledge a like obligation to Dr. Arlidge, and Dr. Langdon Down, — to the latter for his interesting account of the origin and present state of the Asylum for Idiots at Earlswood, and to the former for a valuable notice of the present state of establishments for the treatment of the insane throughout Europe and in the Colonies, and for his assistance on various occasions. To Dr. Arthur Mitchell, I am still more largely indebted for an able notice of Dr. Conolly's writings, as well as for his valuable assistance and advice in reference to many parts of the Memoir.

My best thanks are likewise due to Dr.

Conolly's valued friend and colleague at Hanwell, Dr. Hitchman, for enabling me to fill up
an interesting period of Dr. Conolly's asylum-
life, and for useful information on many points.
To Dr. Conolly's personal friends, Dr. W. A. F.
Browne, Sir Charles Hood, Dr. Bucknill, and
Dr. C. A. Lockhart Robertson, my thanks are
due, for the friendly manner with which they
supplied me with information, which I should
have found a difficulty in obtaining elsewhere.
Indeed, from Dr. Conolly's numerous friends I
always found the greatest readiness to give me
any information which they possessed; and in
giving it, they generally expressed their pleasure
that his merits and labours were to be again
brought before the public.

I must not omit to acknowledge my obligation to Sir James Coxe and Mr. Wilkes for their
important notes showing the extent to which
non-restraint is actually carried out in the existing asylums of England and Scotland; nor those
I owe to my friend Sir Joseph Oliffe for the
trouble he took in procuring for me information regarding the new asylums established in
the vicinity of Paris; and I have still the pleasant duty of expressing my thanks to Dr. Edward

Jarvis for an account of the state of lunacy and of lunatic establishments in the United States. It is gratifying to read Dr. Jarvis's philanthropic and enlightened views as to the treatment of the insane, and to hear of the influence which Dr. Conolly's writings have exercised in promoting the humane treatment of the insane in America.

My own part in the preparation of the Memoir has been a very agreeable one. I can honestly say it has been a labour of love. My long and pleasant friendship with Dr. Conolly, and my natural desire to do justice to his memory, were sufficient incentives to make me undertake the task. As I proceeded with it, the hope arose that by recalling attention to Dr. Conolly's labours in establishing non-restraint, and to the happy results which, in this country, have crowned those labours, the Memoir might have some influence in promoting the extension of the system to other countries. This hope induced me to go more fully into the subject of non-restraint than I had originally intended, and led me to make large extracts from Dr. Conolly's works. I cherish the belief, however, that the history and benefits of that humane

and enlightened treatment of lunacy which he
introduced—told chiefly in his own eloquent
words—will interest every reader who sympa-
thises in efforts to ameliorate the condition of
the insane, whose deplorable lot may be that
of any of us,—for to this greatest of human
calamities all are liable.

If what is said in this Memoir should happily
lead to a fuller adoption of Dr. Conolly's views
by foreign physicians, it will be the realisation
of a hope, which has stimulated me to extend
and complete, what friendship and admiration
led me to think of beginning.

CONTENTS.

—◦◦◦—

I.

II.

III.

IV.

V.

VI.

VII.

VIII.

IX.

X.

XI.

XII.

XIII.

b

XIV.

[1] See Appendix, p. 249.

XVIII.

XIX.

XX.

CONCLUSION.

In preparation of this Memoir, Dr. Conolly's own language used as much as possible in describing his labours—Completion of his benevolent work greatly due to his self-abnegation, kindly disposition, and great consideration for his fellow-labourers—His success shown in the rapid abandonment of mechanical restraint —Subject at times to a desponding state of mind—This led him to fear lest a reaction might interfere with his labours—His

——oo♦oo——

APPENDIX.

MEMOIR

JOHN CONOLLY, M.D., D.C.L.

I.

DR. JOHN CONOLLY, the subject of the following memoir, was an eminent and accomplished physician, distinguished more especially in that branch of the profession with which his name is so intimately associated.

Even before his residence at the University, he had evinced a strong predilection for the study of psychology, and he chose *Insanity* as the subject of his inaugural thesis.[1] After practising for nine years as a general physician, Dr. Conolly directed his whole attention to mental diseases, actuated in a great measure by an ardent desire to ameliorate the condition and improve the treatment of the insane, and more especially of the inmates of our pauper asylums. The success which attended his earnest and persevering efforts in this direction forms the most interesting portion of the following memoir.

[1] *Dissertatio Inauguralis de statu mentis in Insania et Melancholia.*

B

Dr. Conolly was born at Market Rasen, Lincolnshire, in 1794. His father, a younger son of a good Irish family, died early in life. His mother, who was left a widow with a young family, belonged to a respectable county family of the name of Tennyson, and seems to have been a lady of good sense and cultivated mind. Dr. Conolly often spoke of her, and always with great affection and respect. In a letter to a friend he writes, "I cannot now—even now when my own years are declining—reflect on my mother's care when I was young, her patience, her forbearance, and her self-sacrifices, without emotion. I think of her every day of my life, and feel more and more how much of whatever little good has ever been in me was owing to her."

Dr. Conolly was sent at an early age to be educated at the Grammar School of Hedon, of which the vicar of the parish was master. During the seven years which he passed at this school, he learned almost nothing. In some notes on his parentage and education found among his papers, he gives the following account of his early education :—

"For seven years of school life at Hedon, my daily life, except in holidays of three weeks at Midsummer and Christmas, was unvaried. Before nine in the morning I repaired to the school-house. At nine the schoolmaster's awful figure appeared round the corner near the church, and on his entrance I exhibited Latin exercises, written the evening before, and repeated a page or more of the Eton grammar, and construed a portion of whatever Latin author I was advanced to, or of the Greek testament. Between eleven and twelve I construed a second lesson. At noon there were two hours unemployed, except by a frugal dinner and more abundant play. In the afternoon more construing lessons, or, once in the week, a writing copy and some arithmetic. In all these years my schoolmaster, the vicar, never, that I remember, gave me any assistance, except by blows on the head. I read in the usual order, 'Cornelius Nepos,' a book or two of 'Cæsar's Commentaries,' and was then promoted into poetical reading, and at the returning holidays was enabled to inform my few inquiring friends that I was in Ovid and Virgil, and latterly in Horace. Of the absurdity of such reading nothing need be said. I read with difficulty and understood nothing. I was not allowed to read an English lesson. Of the Latin authors I remained profoundly ignorant, never, I believe, except on two occasions, having even a glimmering of their meaning; one being when rather interested with the structure of a bridge over the Rhine, and another when rather excited by the catastrophe of Phaeton, on which latter occasion the exuberance of my feelings was promptly rebuked." [1]

On quitting school he went to reside at Hull with his mother, who had married a second time, her husband being a French gentleman, a political émigré. He went to school at Hull, and was also taught French by his stepfather, who is said to have been very fond of

---

[1] In after life Dr. Conolly became a good classical scholar, and wrote Latin with some elegance.

young Conolly, and not only taught him the language
thoroughly, but made him familiar with some of the
best French authors. This seems to have given
Conolly that taste for French literature which he retained through life. In a letter to his friend M. Battel,
he says, "My thoughts revert more and more to my
earlier days and to my education in your language, to
which I am largely indebted." In another letter he
writes:—"When I am ill and tranquil, I have a
singular pleasure in reading French. The language
is associated in my mind with the early days of my
life and my earliest studies. Condillac's Essai 'Sur
l'Origine des Connaissances Humaines' is now on my
table,—the very volume put into my hands forty years
ago, and of which I seem to remember every word:
perhaps to it I owe the direction of my mental life."

Dr. Conolly entered life at the age of eighteen as an
officer in a militia regiment, in which he served for
several years. He married, while still very young, the
daughter of Sir John Collins, and went to reside in
France, on the banks of the Loire. A year afterwards
he decided on entering the medical profession, and in
1817 began the study of medicine in the University of
Edinburgh, and at the termination of the *curriculum*
received the degree of Doctor of Medicine. He was
much esteemed by his fellow-students at the University,
and was an active member and one of the presidents of
the Royal Medical Society. It was in the discussions
of this Society, and in the essays he wrote for it, that
Dr. Conolly first showed his powers of public speaking

and writing; gifts which he possessed in no ordinary
degree, and which proved so valuable to him in promoting the humane and philanthropic objects in which
he was engaged through the principal part of his life ;
and more especially did they aid him in his labours in
the cause of the lunatic and the imbecile.

Soon after leaving Edinburgh, Dr. Conolly settled in
practice as a physician in Chichester, about the same
time with the late Sir John Forbes. Drawn together
by congenial tastes and pursuits, these two young
physicians formed a warm and life-long friendship, to
which they owed much of their mutual happiness, being
often engaged in similar literary pursuits, or in the interchange of friendly support, when it was the object of
either to promote some public scheme of usefulness or
philanthropy. It was soon found, however, that even
the cathedral town of Chichester did not afford a sufficient field for the practice of two active physicians,
and Dr. Conolly removed to Stratford-on-Avon, where
he remained till 1827, when he was appointed Professor
of the Practice of Medicine in University College,
London.

His residence at Stratford seems to have been one
of the happiest periods of Dr. Conolly's checkered life.
Much of his time was pleasantly occupied in literary
work, and he had a large and agreeable correspondence
with men of science and literature, arising in a great
degree from his connection with the *Society for the Diffusion of Useful Knowledge*, the meetings of which he
generally attended, and to which he contributed various

publications. He was also much engaged in literary
works with his friend Sir John Forbes, chiefly in preparing the *Cyclopædia of Practical Medicine*, a large
and important work, and in editing the *British and
Foreign Medical Review.*

Dr. Conolly took a warm interest in everything that
related to the social condition and sanitary improvements of the borough. He was for several years one of
the aldermen, and served once as mayor. By his own
exertions chiefly, he established a public dispensary,
which proved a great benefit to the poor of Stratford
and the vicinity. And as long as he remained at Stratford he performed gratuitously the duties of physician,
visiting the sick poor at their own homes when they
were unable to come to the dispensary; and he continued to take a warm interest in the prosperity of the
institution long after leaving the place. One source of
his attachment to Stratford was its being the birthplace
of Shakspeare, of whose works he was an ardent student.
In his walks about Stratford, a friend writes me, he
invariably carried a volume of Shakspeare's plays or
sonnets in his pocket, to read in some sequestered spot,
which he imagined Shakspeare himself might have fre-
quented. Writing to his friend Mr. Hunt, in 1861, he
says :—" It is now just thirty-eight years since I settled
at Stratford—often afterwards to be unsettled, until I
found my proper place as friend and guide to the
crazy—and I remember everybody and every circumstance as if it were but yesterday."

He was very popular and much esteemed at Stratford; and, on his appointment to a professorship in the London University, carried with him the grateful remembrance and good wishes of the inhabitants of the town and neighbourhood. Dr. Conolly's professional income at Stratford is said not to have exceeded 400*l.* a year, but my informant added that had he remained he would soon have obtained a large professional income.

In 1835, when residing in Warwick, after he had resigned his professorship in University College, he still interested himself in Stratford, and exerted himself successfully to secure the preservation of Shakspeare's tomb, and the restoration of the chancel of the church. He drew up an appeal to the public for funds, and acted as chairman of the committee formed for this object.

II.

Dr. Conolly's appointment as Professor of the Practice of Medicine, the principal medical chair .in the College, was a remarkable distinction, as he was at that time only *thirty-three* years of age. He held the professorship for nearly four years; but finding that the life of a London physician was not in accordance with his feelings, he resigned the chair and returned to the country, taking up his residence at Warwick, being appointed at the same time Visiting Physician of the Lunatic Asylums in that county, an appointment which he had held when he resided at Stratford.

While professor in University College, Dr. Conolly's thoughts seemed to have been much occupied with the treatment of the insane, and the necessity of insanity forming an essential part of the education of every medical man. With this view he proposed to the Council of the College to give his pupils clinical instruction on insanity, in one of the lunatic asylums in London. His offer was declined, and thus clinical instruction in mental diseases was thrown back for thirty years in this country. About this time he published his work on the *Indications of Insanity*.

He continued to practise at Warwick, with the exception of one year at Birmingham, till 1839, when he was appointed Resident Physician to the Middlesex County Asylum at Hanwell, then the largest in England. Dr. Conolly now felt himself in the position which he had long desired. An ample field was opened to him to put into practice his enlightened and benevolent views on the treatment of the insane, a subject on which he had long meditated; and it may be truly said that after entering on his duty, he did not lose a single day in commencing his mild and humane treatment, so promptly did he make the *total abolition of all mechanical restraint* in Hanwell Asylum a practical fact; thus establishing in that large asylum the most important change ever introduced in the treatment of the insane.

Before entering on Dr. Conolly's system of treatment, it may be interesting to take a brief survey of the origin and progress of the remarkable and beneficial change effected in the treatment of the insane since the conclusion of the last century.

The benevolent and courageous French physician, *Pinel*, was the first to attempt the restoration of the insane to a position among human beings. The scene of his exertions, which formed the first great step towards the non-restraint system, was the *Bicêtre* hospital in Paris for male lunatics. In this frightful hospital, or rather prison, the universal practice was to load patients with heavy chains, often only removed at death, and to immure them in dark, unwarmed, and unventilated cells. Pinel, after full con-

sideration, determined at once to release a large
number of patients. The following account of the
experiment is extracted from the ' British and Foreign
Medical Review :'—

"Towards the end of 1792, Pinel, after having many
times urged the Government to allow him to unchain
the maniacs of the Bicêtre, but in vain, went himself
to the authorities, and with much earnestness and
warmth advocated the removal of this monstrous
abuse. Couthon, a member of the commune, gave
way to M. Pinel's arguments and agreed to meet him
at the Bicêtre. Couthon then interrogated those who
were chained, but the abuse he received, and the con-
fused sounds, cries, vociferations, and clanking of chains
in the filthy and damp cells, made him recoil from
Pinel's proposition. ' You may do what you please with
them,' said he; ' but I fear you will become their
victim.' Pinel instantly commenced his undertaking.
There were about fifty lunatics whom he considered
might without danger to the others be unchained,
and he began by releasing twelve, with the sole pre-
caution of having previously prepared the same number
of strong waistcoats with long sleeves, which could be
tied behind the back, if necessary. The first man on
whom the experiment was to be tried was an English
captain, whose history no one knew, as he had been
in chains forty years. He was thought to be one of
the most furious among them; his keepers approached
him with caution, as he had in a fit of fury killed one
of them on the spot with a blow from his manacles.

He was chained more rigorously than any of the others. Pinel entered his cell unattended, and calmly said to him, 'Captain, I will order your chains to be taken off, and give you liberty to walk in the court, if you will promise me to behave well and injure no one.' 'Yes, I promise you,' said the maniac; 'but you are laughing at me; you are all too much afraid of me.' 'I have six men,' answered Pinel, 'ready to enforce my commands, if necessary. Believe me then, on my word, I will give you liberty if you will put on this waistcoat.' He submitted to this willingly, without a word; his chains were removed, and the keepers retired, leaving the door of the cell open. He raised himself many times from the seat, but fell again on it, for he had been in a sitting posture so long that he had lost the use of his legs; in a quarter of an hour he succeeded in maintaining his balance, and with tottering steps came to the door of his dark cell. His first look was at the sky, and he exclaimed enthusiastically, 'How beautiful!' During the rest of the day he was constantly in motion, walking up and down the staircases, and uttering exclamations of delight. In the evening he returned of his own accord to his cell, where a better bed than he had been accustomed to had been prepared for him, and he slept tranquilly. During the two succeeding years which he spent in the Bicêtre, he had no return of his previous paroxysms, but even rendered himself useful, by exercising a kind of authority over the insane patients, whom he ruled in his own fashion. In the course of

a few days Pinel released fifty-three maniacs from their
chains, among them were men of all conditions and
countries ; workmen, merchants, soldiers, lawyers, &c.
The result was beyond his hopes, tranquillity and harmony succeeded to tumult and disorder, and the whole
discipline was marked with a regularity and kindness
which had the most favourable effect on the insane
themselves, rendering even the most furious more
tractable."

Pinel was a man of talent and extensive acquire-
ments, and of a most benevolent and energetic character. The melancholy loss of a young friend, who
had become insane from excessive mental work in 1783,
first turned Pinel's attention to the study of insanity ;
and it was from his known acquaintance with the
subject, which he had long studied in a private asylum
in Paris, and from his benevolent character, that he
was selected as the physician in Paris best qualified to
take charge of the Bicêtre Lunatic Hospital, at that
time in a state of frightful disorder. Pinel did not
decide to loosen the chains of the lunatics without well
considering the mode of carrying his plan into effect.
He had numerous conversations with *Pussin*, the director
of the Hospital, an uneducated, but sensible, worthy
man, who entered fully into Pinel's views: he also
talked to such of the discontented lunatics as could
understand him, and promised to satisfy their reasonable wants. Pinel thus laid his plans with judgment,
and was rewarded with remarkable success. But this
act of benevolence nearly cost him his life. It was

spread abroad that he had some sinister motive in releasing the lunatics. Under this impression, a furious mob seized him one day, calling " *à la lanterne ;* " and they would probably have carried their intention into effect, but for the exertions of Chevinge, an old soldier of the French Guard, who rescued him from their hands and saved his life. This man was one of those very lunatics in the Bicêtre, who had been liberated by Pinel, afterwards cured, and ultimately taken into his service.[1]

To *Pinel,* therefore, belongs the merit of being the first to abolish chains, and introduce the humane treatment of the Insane, at a time when lunatics throughout the whole of Europe were treated more like wild beasts than human beings. Esquirol, the pupil and friend of Pinel, succeeded him as Physician to the Bicêtre, and was indefatigable in carrying out the philanthropic and enlightened views of his master, both in his practice and by his writings.

The result of Pinel's bold experiment, and his humane treatment in the Bicêtre, produced a strong impression in this country, and the more so, as the public had been recently shocked by the disclosures of the neglect and cruelties practised in the *old* York Asylum. A general feeling of sympathy was excited throughout the kingdom in behalf of the unfortunate and maltreated lunatic, which soon gave rise to a searching enquiry into the condition of our lunatic asylums and the treat-

[1] Pinel: a Biographical Study, by his nephew, Dr. Casimir Pinel.

ment of their inmates. The consequence was a great improvement in both. This feeling in favour of the insane continued, and ultimately resulted, chiefly by the efforts of Conolly, in the total abolition of all mechanical restraint in the treatment of the insane.

While Pinel was loosening the chains of the lunatic in the *Bicêtre*, William Tuke was quietly establishing the *Retreat* near York, which came into full operation in 1796.[1] "Of this admirable asylum," writes Dr. Conolly, "the first in Europe in which every enlightened principle of treatment was carried into effect, the chief promoter was the late William Tuke of York."[2]

This formed the first step in this country towards an improved treatment of the insane : the next step was the total disuse of mechanical restraints, first adopted by the late Dr. Charlesworth and Mr. Gardiner Hill, in Lincoln Asylum. While non-restraint was being quietly practised in this small asylum, Dr. Conolly was appointed Resident Physician to the Middlesex County Asylum at Hanwell (1839), and he at once proceeded to abolish all mechanical restraint in that asylum, containing upwards of 800 patients, "being satisfied," he

---

[1] The establishment of the *Retreat*, Dr. Thurnum writes, was by a singular and interesting coincidence proposed in the spring of 1792, the very year in which Pinel gave the first blow to restraint.— Prize Essay, by Daniel Tuke, M.D. It is a matter of no essential consequence, but it appears in a notice of Pinel's life by his nephew, Dr. Casimir Pinel, that his appointment to the Bicêtre Hospital was in "the latter end of 1793 and not in 1792."—Casimir Pinel, *Journal of Psychological Medicine*, vol. xiii.

[2] *Treatment of the Insane*, p. 17.

said, " from what he had witnessed in Lincoln Asylum,
that mechanical restraint was not only unnecessary, but
possibly injurious."

Dr. Conolly's appointment to the Hanwell Asylum
at this time was a most fortunate circumstance for the
progress of the non-restraint system. It had then
taken so little hold of the professional mind, indeed
was so little known, owing to the quiet manner in
which it had been conducted in the Lincoln Asylum,
that but for Dr. Conolly's having been placed in a
position to carry it out practically on a large scale,
under the eyes of the profession, and even of the public,
it might have lapsed into neglect, and its beneficial
effects have been lost for years, as another physician
possessed of the energy, the perseverance, and enthu-
siasm of Conolly was not likely soon to be found. Even
with his rare qualities, we shall see that he had great
difficulties to contend with, and obstacles to overcome
during a struggle of many years, to ensure for non-
restraint a broad and full success.

To *Pinel* in France, therefore, and to *Tuke* in England, may be justly ascribed the honour of being the
first to introduce the mild and humane treatment of the
insane ; to Dr. Charlesworth and Mr. Hill, that of being
the first to adopt *non-restraint ;* while to Dr. Conolly
belongs the merit, as we shall presently see, of demonstrating that non-restraint is perfectly practicable in
every asylum. M. Battel, an eminent French physician, fully acquainted with the subject of non-restraint,
has expressed in the following simple terms the re-

spective merits of Pinel and Conolly in originating and establishing the non-restraint system :—

" Notre célèbre Pinel est devenu l'une de nos illustrations pour avoir fait tomber les chaines des aliénés. Mais il n'avait accompli que la moitié la moins difficile de la tâche, et Conolly ne sera pas moins illustre pour avoir supprimé les entraves et tous les indignes moyens de coercition." [1]

Dr. Conolly, by his judicious and energetic conduct while Resident Physician to the Hanwell Asylum, succeeded in establishing *non-restraint* as the invariable practice in that institution, and in satisfying the numerous members of the medical profession who visited Hanwell, in order to witness the practice carried out under his direction, not only of its perfect safety, but of its happy influence in calming the most excited lunatics, and of its tranquillising effects throughout the whole asylum.

The fame of the non-restraint system of treatment at Hanwell led to the asylum being visited by physicians, and particularly by the medical superintendents of asylums both of this and other countries. One of these was M. Battel, Inspector-General of Civil Hospitals in Paris, who was commissioned officially to examine into the Hanwell treatment and its results. After careful observation of the whole system, M. Battel returned to Paris a warm advocate of non-restraint. Unfortunately he failed to induce his colleagues to form the same opinion of it. This visit led to the formation of a warm

[1] Letter to the author of this Memoir.

friendship between M. Battel and Dr. Conolly, which did not cease till the death of the latter, an intimate correspondence having been kept up the whole time. M. Battel, in a letter to myself, gives the following account of his visit, and of the friendship it led to, a friendship honourable to the character of both:—

"Le Conseil Général de mon administration avait entendu parler du nouvel asile de Hanwell, de ses heureuses installations, de son excellente direction et des soins éclairés qu'y recevaient les pauvres aliénés; il me chargea de le visiter. Cette mission me mit en rapport avec Conolly, et je me la rappelle toujours comme l'une des plus heureuses circonstances de ma vie. Son esprit élevé, les sentiments généreux qu'il professait, sa douceur, son humanité, m'inspirèrent aussitôt pour lui la plus vive et la plus profonde sympathie. Nos relations constantes depuis cette époque et la conformité de nos idées, établirent entre nous une étroite amitié, dont le souvenir me sera toujours précieux, parce que je la considère comme ayant été l'un des principaux honneurs de ma vie."

The publication also of Dr. Conolly's admirable *Annual Reports* on the progress of the system, made its beneficial effects generally known to all who felt an interest in the treatment of the insane. Nothing can exceed the clear and simple manner in which he describes in these Reports the treatment year by year, and refutes the groundless accusations which were made against it by its enemies.

"The first four of these Annual Reports, those

C

namely for 1839, 1840, 1841, and 1842," we are told
by Dr. Robertson, in his late Presidential Address to
the Medico-Psychological Association (1867), "still
form the groundwork of our treatment of the insane
poor in the English county asylums, while these
asylums themselves—whose fame (I may be permitted
to say), based as it is on the successful application
of the English non-restraint system, has gone forth
into the whole civilized world, and thus brought
rescue to the most suffering and degraded of our
race—stand throughout this fair land imperishable
monuments of the *statesman* to whom they owe their
origin, and of the *physician* who asserted the great
principle on which the treatment within their walls
is founded." [1]

Very rarely indeed do Annual Reports of this character, which in their nature are more or less ephemeral,
acquire and maintain such a reputation and usefulness,
and exercise such a prolonged influence on public and
professional opinion. It is, perhaps, equally rare for a
man to enter on a great scheme of reform, with views
of its basis and scope so clear as to enable him, from
the very outset, to give it a direction which needed no
subsequent change; and to rest its claims on the
very threshold, on reasons so sound and so compre-
hensive, that they gained little in strength by later
experience.

[1] 'The President's Address, 1867, by C. Lockhart Robertson, M.D.
Cantab., Medical Superintendent of the Sussex Lunatic Asylum,
Hayward's Heath,' &c. &c., p. 11.

III.

EVER since the philanthropic *Pinel* abolished the chains and inaugurated the humane treatment of the insane in France, and *William Tuke* established a mild and rational system of treatment in this country, the condition of lunatic asylums throughout a great part of Europe has been undergoing, although slowly, a favourable change, moral means gradually taking the place of physical restraint ; still, I believe, I am correct in stating, that mechanical restraints—chains not always excluded—were freely used in every asylum in Europe, the Bicêtre in Paris, the Lincoln Asylum, and the Retreat in England excepted, when Dr. Conolly was appointed to Hanwell Asylum. Nor did Hanwell form an exception to the general practice : for, although under the direction of Sir William and Lady Ellis a comparatively mild treatment had been adopted, and the system of employing as many of the patients as possible in agricultural and other occupations had been introduced—although, in consequence of these improvements, Hanwell was deservedly considered one of the best managed asylums in England; nevertheless, when Dr. Conolly assumed the direction, one year after Sir W. Ellis had resigned, "instruments of mechanical restraint, of one kind or other, were so abundant in the wards as to amount, when collected together, to

c 2

about six hundred, half of them being handcuffs and
leg-locks."[1]

Dr. Conolly entered on his duties as Resident Physician at Hanwell Asylum, on the 1st of June, 1839,
the Asylum at that time containing 800 patients, of
whom he found over forty under mechanical restraint;
and in his *First Report* to the Quarter Sessions, on 31st
October, 1839, he states that since the 21st of September not one patient in the asylum had been under
restraint. He adds,—" no form of strait-waistcoat, no
handcuffs, no leg-locks, nor any contrivance confining
the trunk, or limbs, or any of the muscles, is now in
use. The coercion chairs, about forty in number, have
been altogether removed from the wards." The reasons
for making so great a change in the discipline of the
Asylum are given in the following extract from the
Report :—

" The article of treatment which the Resident Physician has thought it expedient to depart the most
widely from in the previous practice of the Asylum,
has been that which relates to the personal *coercion*
or forcible *restraint* of the refractory patients. Without any intention of derogating from the high character
acquired by the Asylum, it appeared to him that the
advantage resulting from the degree of restraint permitted and customary in it, at the period of his appointment, was in no respect proportionate to the frequency

[1] *Treatment of the Insane,* p. 190.

of its application; that the objections to the restraint
actually employed were very serious; and that it was
in fact creative of many of the outrages and disorders,
to repress which its application was commonly deemed
indispensable, and consequently, directly opposed to the
chief design of all treatment in the cure of the disease.
The example of the Lincoln Asylum, in which no
patient has been put in restraint for nearly three years,
came also powerfully in aid of an attempt to govern
the Asylum at Hanwell by mental restraint rather than
by physical."

Such is the essential part of Dr. Conolly's First
Report, which recorded the fact, that in the space of
four months the use of all forms of mechanical restraint
had been abandoned in an asylum, with a population
of 800 lunatics, and gave reasons for the change of
treatment, which are the same as those we should still
use if we were advocating such a reform. This work,
it deserves remark, was accomplished by a physician
who had never before been in charge of an asylum.
It deserves remark, also, that Dr. Conolly availed himself of the first opportunity that offered, to acknowledge
the extent to which his views had been influenced by
the success of the treatment pursued in the Lincoln
Asylum.

The following letter, written at this time to his friend
Mr. Hunt of Stratford, expresses perhaps more fully
than a formal Report, how Dr. Conolly's mind was
bound up in his work, and how firm was his resolve to
carry it through :—

"I know you will be glad to hear that we have now ruled this great house for four months without a single instance of restraint by any of the old and objectionable methods. The use of strait-waistcoats is abolished; hand-straps and leg-locks are never resorted to; and the restraint chairs have been cut up to make a floor for the carpenter's shop. All this has, of course, occasioned some trouble and some anxiety; but the success of the plan, and its visible good effects, abundantly repay me. I think I feel more deeply interested in my work every day. I meet with the most constant and kind support of the magistrates; indeed, my only fear is that they should say too much of what is done here, and thus provoke enmity and censure.

Our asylum is now almost daily visited by the officers of other institutions, who are curious to know what method of restraint we *do* resort to; and they can scarcely believe that we rely wholly on constant superintendence, constant kindness, and firmness when required."

No one will read this short note without interest and pleasure. It reveals that earnest benevolence which stimulated Dr. Conolly to meet and conquer the difficulties which he knew awaited him. And it reveals also in a few sentences the complete enlightenment of his views, when he first undertook that work, the accomplishment of which has made him so famous.

The following brief notice of the *History* of non-

restraint in Hanwell Asylum is taken from Dr. Conolly's
'Extracts from his Annual Reports to the Visiting
Magistrates, from 1839 to 1849.' These extracts are
abridged, but they are given in Dr. Conolly's own
words, and it is hoped they will be found sufficient to
show the working and success of the system. The
original Reports were illustrated by cases and by
remarks on various points connected with the management of the Asylum, most of which are also given
in Dr. Conolly's extracts in his work on the *Treatment
of the Insane without Restraint.* The Reports themselves, which cannot now be obtained in their complete
form, were made when the non-restraint system was in
progress, and were read with eagerness by all interested
in the welfare of the insane.

In his *Second Report*, 1840, Dr. Conolly was able
to announce that there had been no return to the use
of mechanical restraint in any form.

"During the past year," he says, "not one instance
has occurred in which the Resident Physician has
thought it advisable to resort to any of the forms of
bodily coercion formerly employed. Nine suicidal
cases are among the admissions of this year, and it
affords gratification to the Physician to be enabled to
state, that in all these cases means have been found
to sooth and comfort the minds of the patients, and
apparently to reconcile them to life. Their restraints
have been in all cases immediately removed, and in
no case resorted to again. They have been watched

so long as it was deemed necessary, during the day, placed in rooms with other patients by night, and frequently visited. Every instrument of danger, or obvious means of self-destruction, has been kept out of their way ; and no measure likely to restore cheerfulness has been omitted. This is the general plan resorted to. But in almost every case of this kind the bodily health is manifestly disordered ; and when proper remedial measures are applied the propensity to suicide is weakened, or disappears."

There appears to have been a dread that it would be found impossible to abstain from restraint in the case of suicidal patients, and in his second Report, we find Dr. Conolly showing this fear, like all others, to be groundless.

Dr. Hitchman, on the same point, after describing the intense anxiety produced by the care and treatment of suicidal patients, remarks, "It is among the bright results of that treatment which Charlesworth and Hill conceived, and which the genius of a Conolly expounded and confirmed, that it tends to diminish the suicidal impulse, by removing the sense of degradation which restraints involve, and by surrounding the patients with cheerful influences and bringing them more completely under medical control."[1]

In his *Third Report*, 1841, Dr. Conolly says,— "More than two years have now been completed since

[1] *Annual Reports of County Lunatic Asylums*, 1856.

the Resident Physician began to report to the Visiting
Justices the gradual disuse of all mechanical modes
of restraint, and the substitution of a more efficient
superintendence by means of a greater number of attendants of intelligence and respectability." The
motives for the reform in treatment, as he then gave
them, "were the apparent inefficacy of mechanical
restraint as a means of preventing accidents and mischief; its irritating effects on the violent; the alarm it
occasioned to the timid; and its tendency to debase
those to whom, and by whom it was applied, and to
create incurable habits of uncleanliness."

In this Report also he thus states the result of his
experience of the effects of restraint on refractory
patients:—
  "The Physician speaks from repeated observation,
when he says, that no favourable impression could
be made upon these patients, so long as restraints were
either resorted to, or threatened. Yet in these patients
the mere mention of restraint was often observed to
cause the patient's face to become deadly pale, an evidence
of its efficacy as a punishment: standing quite apart
from any proof of its efficacy as a means of moral
control. The spectacle, in these cases, when the strait-
waistcoat was determined upon, was most distressing.
There was a violent struggle; the patient was overcome by main force; the limbs were secured by the
attendants, with a tightness proportioned to the difficulty they had encountered, and the patient was left,

heated, irritated, mortified, and probably bruised and
hurt, without one consoling word : left to scream, to
shout, to execrate, and apparently to exhaust the whole
soul in bitter and hateful expressions, and in curses too
horrible for human ears. It was impossible to view
these things almost daily occurring without resolving
to endeavour to prevent them." Dr. Conolly concludes
this Report by recording the high opinion he entertained of the value of the services of his matron. "I
cannot close my Report," he says, "without recording
as a means enabling me in a great measure to disregard some of the difficulties to which I have alluded,
the constant support which my efforts have received
from Miss Powell, the Matron, whose daily and hourly
services, have been, and are, such as I shall not attempt
to characterize, except by saying that they are incal-
culable, although from their very nature, many of them
are known to few earthly witnesses."

This is not the only occasion on which Dr. Conolly
expresses his obligations and thanks to his excellent
matron for her valuable and unceasing exertions in
enabling him to carry out the non-restraint system.

The three *Reports* presented by Dr. Conolly in 1839,
1840, and 1841, contain many details of a system
adopted by him from the Lincoln Asylum, and persevered in with such modifications as experience suggested, to dispense in the treatment of the insane with
all bodily restraints. In his *Fourth Report*, 1842, he
says that he " has now only the agreeable task of re-

cording that time, and patience, and the zealous co-operation of all the officers of the Asylum, have enabled him to overcome many obstacles, and have confirmed him in the belief, at first encouraged with much diffidence, but now established beyond the likelihood of ever being overthrown, that the management of a large asylum is not only practicable without the application of bodily coercion to the patients, *but that, after the total disuse of such a method of control, the whole character of an asylum undergoes a gradual and beneficial change.*"

The *Fifth Report*, 1843, reiterates all that was said in former Reports as to the good effects of non-restraint in simplifying the management of an asylum.

"The whole experience of the last twelve months," he says, "has fully confirmed the impression, made in the years preceding, that by the abolition of physical restraints the general management of the insane has been freed from many difficulties, and their recovery in various degrees greatly promoted. Fresh illustrations have been daily afforded of the advantage of those general principles of treatment which have been expressed in former Reports; and of which the effects are to remove, as far as possible, all causes of irritation and excitement from the irritable; to soothe, encourage, and comfort the depressed; to repress the violent by methods which leave no ill effect on the temper, and leave no painful recollections in the memory; and, in all cases, to seize every opportunity of promoting a

restoration of the healthy exercise of the understanding
and of the affections." . . .

" Insanity, thus treated, undergoes great if not unex-
pected modifications; and the wards of lunatic asylums
no longer illustrate the harrowing description of their
former state. Mania, not exasperated by severity and
melancholia, not deepened by the want of all ordinary
consolations, lose the exaggerated character in which
they were formerly beheld. Hope takes the place of
fear, severity is substituted for discontent, and the mind
is left in a condition favourable to every impression
likely to call forth salutary efforts."

In this Report Dr. Conolly points to the remarkable
effect of the absence of restraint in removing all causes
of irritation and excitement, and in modifying mental
diseases, so that they lose the exaggerated character in
which they were formerly beheld, and thus become more
amenable to treatment.

The quotation which follows, from the *Sixth Report*,
1844, is one of special value, as it refers to those measures which are resorted to, or are said to be resorted
to, as substitutes for restraint.

" Five years having now been completed since the
abolition of every form of mechanical restraint, without
the occurrence of any accident which the ordinary application of such modes of restraint could have prevented,
and with a marked improvement in the character of
those parts of the Asylum in which restraints were in
continual use, I should not think it necessary to say

more on this subject than that my confidence in the practicability, safety, and advantages of the non-restraint system has gained strength by every year's experience since September, 1839; if I did not observe that much misconception still exists concerning the substitutes for restraints, in consequence of which doubts continue to be entertained, by many whose opinions must always have considerable weight, respecting the real advantage of this mode of treatment.

" The principal error is that of confounding the idea of temporary seclusion in ordinary sleeping rooms with solitary confinement.

" Seclusion, as directed to be practised in Hanwell, is but the removal of a patient from a gallery to a quiet bed-room opening directly out of the gallery; from noise and excitement to tranquillity. It is only resorted to when the patient cannot be at large with safety to himself or to others, and when he is not in a state to be influenced by persuasion, or conciliated by kindness; and it is only continued until the temporary passion has subsided and the danger is past. In extreme cases, the protection of the patient is further secured by his being placed in a room of which the floor is a bed, and the four walls are padded. This room is not always darkened even by the closure of the shutter, and it is never completely dark. The seclusion is immediately reported to the medical officers, and a daily record of every case of seclusion is kept,—even in cases in which it is only continued for half-an-hour, or for a shorter period. There is no single point in the management of the patients at

Hanwell to which I have paid such frequent and anxious
attention, as to seclusion and its effects, immediate and
remote.   Its immediate effect is, of course, to protect
the other patients, or the patient himself, from every
danger; but it also scarcely ever fails to calm the
patient's feelings, and to put a stop to his vociferations
almost as soon as it is carried into effect.   The patient
who was five minutes before filling the gallery or the
air with shouts, and exhausting himself in vehement
and menacing actions, is found at once to cease to shout
and threaten; to walk up and down his room, quickly
at first but soon more quietly; then to sit down and
read, or to lie down and sleep.   Women so secluded will
walk about for a short time, and then take up a needle
and thread and begin to sew.   These effects of seclusion
I continually observe; and the exceptions to them are
most rare."

In this extract from his Sixth Report, Dr. Conolly
deals with a point of some importance.   As might have
been expected, doubts were entertained by many when
the non-restraint system was promulgated, as to its real
efficiency, and it was thought and even asserted by some
foreign alienist physicians, that restraint had found a
substitute in seclusion.   This error Dr. Conolly takes
pains to correct, and what he has said on the subject
may still prove useful, since the same error and misconception prevail to a considerable degree on the continent
at the present day.   The limited and judicious manner
in which Dr. Conolly used seclusion, is a sufficient

refutation of the groundless assertion as to its improper use in Hanwell.

From the *Seventh Report*, 1845:—" Without making further allusion to the subject of restraint, I shall on this occasion merely observe that the sixth year, during which the great experiment of managing every kind of case without having recourse to it by day or by night, has been completed without the occurrence of any accident which restraint could have effectually prevented, and without the occurrence of any suicide; and that the non-restraint system appears to be becoming gradually adopted in a greater number of asylums, both public and private."

To be able to write the last three lines of this extract must have been very gratifying to Dr. Conolly.

From the *Eighth Report*, 1846:—" On the 21st day of September last, seven years were completed, during which no means of mechanical restraint have been resorted to in the Hanwell Asylum, by night or by day. In those seven years, 1100 cases have been admitted, and treated entirely on the non-restraint system; and the number of patients in the Asylum has, during a great part of the same period, amounted to nearly 1000.

" In the Annual Reports of past years, when the experiment was but in an early stage of its progress, and when it was embarrassed by many difficulties, I refrained from engaging in any controversy on the subject; being satisfied that the results would furnish the best test of its being rational and judicious, as well as humane. If such results had not appeared, it would have been my duty to modify or abandon the system, as, in similar circumstances, it would have been my duty to alter or relinquish any other particular in the treatment of the patients. . . . Now, after seven years' patient trial, during which the non-restraint system has been introduced into many other asylums, without the occurrence of any accident against which mechanical restraint would have afforded security, I do not think it desirable to notice more particularly the opinions of writers who have sometimes appeared to visit Hanwell more prepared to argue than disposed to observe; nor should I deem it necessary to refer to this part of the treatment, if it were not that I consider it still requisite to remind those who are most anxious to adopt it, that certain conditions are essential to its being successfully maintained.

"One of the first of these is, a properly constructed building, in which the patients enjoy the advantages of light and air, and a cheerful prospect, and ample space for exercise, and for classification, and means of occupation and recreation. The next is the constant and watchful superintendence of humane and intelligent officers, exercising full but considerate and just control over an efficient body of attendants."

In this his Eighth Report, Dr. Conolly draws attention to the large number of lunatics who had been under treatment during the first seven years after the dis-

appearance of restraint from Hanwell Asylum. He
expresses himself as fully justified in appealing to results
in support of his views in the application of the non-
restraint system to every form of insanity.

In Dr. Conolly's hands the result of non-restraint
was complete, and he admitted of no exception; but a
more extended experience of the system in other hands,
has shown that cases do occasionally occur which cannot
be controlled without the aid of some mechanical assistance. This is even admitted by the warmest advocates
of the system, and may be so without impeaching the
principle of non-restraint; but that such exceptions to
the rule are rare, in well-managed asylums, will be
evident from the fact that, in ten years' practice in an
asylum containing nearly a thousand patients, Dr.
Conolly did not meet one such case. And it will be
seen by a reference to the reports of some of our oldest
medical superintendents, that the exceptions are almost
equally rare as in Conolly's practice at Hanwell.[1]

The *Eleventh Report*, 1849, is the last one which Dr.
Conolly wrote, and it enables him to speak after an
experience of ten years. He says:—" Ten years of
the trial of a system of treatment at the Hanwell
Asylum, from which all methods of mechanical restraint have been strictly excluded, were completed at
the end of the month of September, 1849.

"I will only further simply state, that now, for ten

[1] See Recent Reports of Medical Superintendents of our County
Asylums, p. 161–3.

entire years, no hand or foot has been fastened in this
large Asylum by day or by night, for the control of the
violent or the despairing; that no instrument of
mechanical restraint has been employed, or even admitted into the wards for any reason whatever; that no
patient has been placed in a coercion-chair by day, or
fastened to a bedstead at night ; and that every patient,
however excited or apparently unmanagable, arriving at
the Asylum in restraints, has been immediately set free
and remained so from that time. I wish to overstate
nothing; but I am justified in adding, that the results,
more and more seen in every successive year, have been
increased tranquillity, diminished danger, and so salutary
an influence over the recent and newly-admitted and
most violent cases, as to make the spectacle of the more
terrible forms of mania and melancholia a rare exception
to the general order and cheerfulness of the establishment.

" I must add, for the satisfaction of those who have
ever been led to suppose that severe medical means of
restraint have been rendered necessary, and relied upon
in the absence of restraints, that, among the substitutes
for mechanical restraints, the temporary seclusion of
patients—that salutary exclusion of causes of excitement from an already irritated brain, which has so
unjustly been stigmatised as solitary imprisonment—is
found to be but seldom necessary, except for a few hours,
and as an actual remedy which the soundest principles
of medicine would recognise in every disease of excitement.   The douche-bath is never employed in any case;

and the shower-bath is rarely resorted to, except for medical reasons; whilst window-guards, dresses of very strong materials, strong blanket-cases, and all the inventions required to limit the mischiefs to which many patients are prone, are only required in a proportion of cases very small in relation to the whole. But it ought never to be forgotten that the necessity for such resources must always depend on the character of the officers and attendants in an asylum. The great and only real substitute for restraint is invariable kindness. This feeling must animate every person employed in every duty to be performed."

The summary of these Reports, which Dr. Conolly prepared to illustrate the history and progress of non-restraint from its beginning, concluded in the following impressive words:—

"These Reports were drawn up from observation in each year, of the facts related in them, until at length the experiment seemed complete, and the system established. I am enabled to refer to them with what I hope is a justifiable satisfaction, as I am not conscious of having at any time employed exaggerated expressions in them, or coloured any of the facts they contain, too highly. In them and in my *Clinical Lectures* published in the *Lancet* in 1846, and in my work on the *Construction and Government of Asylums*, published in 1847, the inquirer in the subject of the general treatment of the insane will find the principal results of my experience. To these some future additions may pos-

D 2

sibly be added; but even as they at present appear, I
trust there is nothing to lead the student into error,
or to mislead the practitioner in this department of
medicine."

Dr. Conolly availed himself of his Annual Reports to
the Visiting Magistrates, and on several other opportunities, to express publicly his obligations to the successful labours of Dr. Charlesworth in Lincoln Asylum,
as his great encouragement to introduce non-restraint
at once into Hanwell Asylum. And a few years before
his death he took the occasion of the inauguration of
Dr. Charlesworth's statue to repeat them, with his
opinion of the character of that good man.

" I have been most anxious," he said, "to attend
on the present occasion, not only that I might assist
in the performance of a public duty, but because I
have always acknowledged how large a debt of gratitude I personally owe to Dr. Charlesworth, whose
services in the cause of the insane you are now met
to commemorate. To those services I must confess
myself chiefly indebted for the determination to do
what afterward I had opportunities of effecting in the
same direction. There had been great benefactors to
the insane before Dr. Charlesworth, and he willingly
bore testimony to what they had done. Pinel, in the
stormy time of the first French Revolution, had
liberated many lunatics from chains and dungeons.
The Society of Friends had established the Retreat at
York, where every humane principle in treatment was

carried into practical effect. Still, the state of most of
the asylums of this country remained very defective, and
the condition of the insane very miserable. The York
County Asylum and the great Asylum of Bethlehem
presented deplorable examples of neglect and cruelty at
that time; and in every asylum there were to be found
patients who had been chained and fettered for years—
ill-fed, ill-clothed, and ill-treated in every possible manner. The records of the Lincoln Asylum show that as
early as the year 1821, two years after the opening of
the Institution, Dr. Charlesworth's attention was strongly
directed to the improvement of the treatment of insane
persons. Step by step may be traced in those records
the mitigation of the condition of the patients; the
substitution of various means of security, without the
necessity of resorting to severe mechanical restraints.
Increased liberty was given to them, their superintendence was rendered more efficient, and one by one the
terrible inventions for fastening them up became unnecessary, and were destroyed. It appears to me that it was
Dr. Charlesworth's peculiar merit, and that it constitutes
his peculiar claim to our grateful remembrance, that he
persevered in this great work, year after year, regardless
of opposition, and undaunted by difficulties; and that
he so animated the resident officers of the Asylum that
at length with his superintendence they accomplished
that which perhaps he had scarcely been sanguine
enough to expect, and found that the total abolition of
mechanical restraints was possible, and actually effected
it. This had taken place a short time before I visited

the Lincoln Asylum in May, 1839. I was then about to take the direction of the Hanwell Asylum, and I visited several Institutions to observe what was done in them. I found improvements going on in most of them; but restraints still used in them all—strait-waistcoats, handcuffs, leg-locks, various coarse devices of leather and iron, including gags and horrible screws to force open the mouths of unhappy patients, who were unwilling or even unable to take food. At Lincoln alone I found none of these things. I do not mean to say that I found a perfect system; but I found watching and care substituted for mechanical restraints. From Dr. Charlesworth's lips I afterwards heard an exposition of his views and principles; and I certainly left Lincoln with a hope—almost with a determination—of carrying out those principles which were, I knew, the real principles of Pinel and Samuel Tuke more fully developed. It was my privilege, and has been the happiness of my life, to effect this at Hanwell; and whilst I live I shall always be proud to acknowledge my debt to Lincoln. From September, 1839, to the present time,[1] no hand or foot has been bound at Hanwell by night or by day. In my first printed Report of Hanwell, and on numerous subsequent occasions, my acknowledgments to Lincoln have been fully and gratefully expressed, and I repeat them now before the statue of Dr. Charlesworth, because but for what I saw at Lincoln I might never have thought of what it was afterwards in my power to effect

---

[1] That is during a period of ten years.

on a larger scale at Hanwell. The system of non-restraint has yet its opponents."

It is evident from this speech, and from that which Dr. Conolly delivered on the occasion of a presentation of a testimonial to him, that the safety and propriety of abandoning mechanical restraint in the treatment of the insane, was not one of those accidental discoveries which are occasionally made with little mental effort. On the contrary, it was the fruit of much careful observation and reflection; and the experiment was persevered in amidst difficulties for many years by a man of no ordinary sagacity, firmness of purpose, and benevolence of disposition. Such a man was Dr. Charlesworth, who may be truly called the father of the non-restraint treatment of the lunatic, which it was Dr. Conolly's work to complete and establish on an indestructible basis.

IV.

AFTER holding the appointment of Resident Physician
for ten years, at the termination of which it was found
that the *non-restraint* system was securely established
in Hanwell Asylum, and that it was making great
progress throughout the country, Dr. Conolly was
appointed Visiting Physician; the appointment of Resident Physician having been discontinued. The treatment of the patients in the Asylum was assigned to the
two medical officers, Dr. Hitchman and Dr. Begley,
one having charge of the female and the other of the
male department of the Asylum.

For the following account of Dr. Conolly's attendance as Visiting Physician, I am indebted to Dr. Hitchman, Medical Superintendent to the Derbyshire Asylum,
and the intimate friend of Dr. Conolly :—

"Dr. Conolly visited the Asylum twice a week, spend-
ing the greater portion of the day at each visit. His
interest in the patients seemed never to flag. Even
cases beyond all hope of recovery were still objects of
his attention. He was always pleased to see them
happy, and had a kind word for each. Simple things
which vainer men with less wisdom would have disregarded, or looked upon as too insignificant for their
notice, arrested Dr. Conolly's attention, and supplied

matter for remark and commendation—*e. g.*, a face
cleaner than usual, hair more carefully arranged, a
neater cap, a new riband, clothes put on with greater
neatness, and numerous little things of a like kind,
enabled him to address his poor illiterate patients in
gentle and loving accents, and thus woke up their feeble
minds, caused their sad faces to gleam with a smile,
even though transient, and made his visit to the wards
to be longed for and appreciated. Dr. Conolly rejoiced
in acts of beneficence. To be poor and to be insane were
conditions which at once endeared the sufferers to him ;
and when the insanity was removed, and the patient
left the Asylum, he generally strove to obtain some
pecuniary aid for her from the 'Adelaide Fund' (a
fund originated for the relief of discharged patients),
and supplemented this very often indeed with liberal
donations from his own purse. I believe that he gave
away large sums of money in this manner.

"I was not associated with the Doctor when he first
introduced the non-restraint system ; but the older
attendants of the Asylum, on both sides of the Institution, spoke often to me of his ceaseless vigilance during
the early years of that great experiment—of his visiting
the wards at all hours of the night, and frequently more
than once, walking noiselessly along the corridors in
slippers specially made for this purpose, thus keeping
the 'night attendants' to their duty, and ministering
in various ways to the comfort of the restless, sleepless
patients under his care. He was, indeed, a noble en-
thusiast, in the best sense of the term. His work was a

labour of passionate love, and his language, therefore, was often fervid. Thus he wrote to me, ' I feel grateful to God, who has entrusted duties to me which angels might stoop to perform.' He had, however, in common with all men engaged in great duties, his moments of despondency. He was also a great sufferer from an irritable chronic skin affection, which often deprived him of much sleep at night, and irritated him during the day; and this sometimes caused him to appear impatient and excitable by officers and others who knew not or could not appreciate the corporeal conditions and mental anxieties which produced the feeling. He was, in truth, at all times supersensitive, reminding one too frequently of Burns's pathetic lines—

> ' Chords that vibrate sweetest pleasure
> Thrill the deepest notes of woe.'

" I write, *currente calamo*, but I think I have answered briefly all your enquiries. His letters to me refer too much to persons now living to admit of publication,—moreover, many I regard as private and sacred;—but the one he penned to me from his sick chamber, not long prior to his death, was so encouraging to myself, and I think so characteristic of a faithful Christian man, that I cannot forego the pleasure of transcribing its closing sentences for your perusal:—' I hope you and Mrs. Hitchman are well, and free from earthly discomfort, happy I would say in doing no unimportant work. I am free from suffering, and quite resigned to live as long, or to die as soon, as

God pleases; thankful to have lived; truly lamenting
that my life has been so little worthy of the ever good
Giver, but never despairing.'

"'Being dead—he yet speaketh,' not only by his
writings, but in the public lunatic asylums of this and
other lands. His personal reputation, the fulness and
lucidity of his *Hanwell Reports*, and more especially
his practical work, *On the Construction and Government of Lunatic Asylums*, caused him to be much
consulted by county magistrates, architects, and others,
who were contemplating the erection of a lunatic asylum,
and thus he became a great agent in displacing the
gloomy 'Mad-House' of the past, and in supplying
appropriate hospitals for the treatment of the insane.
Dr. Conolly educated the public mind, and taught it to
know that a good house and a pleasant site were *essen-
tials* in the restoration of a disordered mind; and now,
almost every county in England is provided with a
lunatic hospital formed on the general principles advocated by him. These hospitals stand on many a beautiful hill, alike monuments of his fame, and of the
Christian benevolence of the English people.

"The retrospect of Dr. Conolly's friendship is most
pleasing; a friendship never suspended for a passing
moment during the five years we were associated in
office, or indeed, ever afterwards. It was a pleasure
and an honour to know so great and so good a man."

In 1852 Dr. Conolly resigned the appointment of
Visiting Physician, and from that time his connection
with Hanwell Asylum may be said to have ceased;

for although he was appointed Consulting Physician, there were scarcely any duties attached to the office, and he rarely visited Hanwell.

On his retirement, his professional friends presented him with a testimonial in the form of a handsome piece of plate emblematic of the work in which he had been so long engaged, and a portrait of himself by Sir Watson Gordon.

The testimonial was presented by the Earl of Shaftesbury. His Lordship, addressing Dr. Conolly, said :—

"Dr. John Conolly, the gentlemen assembled here this day, your friends and admirers, and I may add, moreover, the representatives of your friends and admirers throughout all parts of this kingdom, have assigned to me the very real honour and the very high gratification of requesting your acceptance of the testimonials now exhibited in this room. We rejoice in the opportunity thus afforded us of testifying the delight and of recording the satisfaction we feel, in witnessing the great progress of science and humanity under your auspices in regard to the treatment of the insane, and that you have been thus selected as an eminent instrument in following out this great work of wisdom and humanity. It would be unbecoming in me to enter into any narrative of the history, or of the results of what is termed the 'non-coercion system.' But to understand thoroughly the remarkable merits of Dr. Conolly, we must remember the state of things which prevailed in lunatic asylums some years ago. Nothing could have been more horrible than the treatment of lunatics some forty

years ago. The lunatic was treated without any regard
to cure, and regarded as a savage beast who was only
to be coerced; and the lunatic asylum was worse than
the prison. Now, all that is changed. Nearly every
vestige of ancient barbarism and ignorance has been
effaced; and soon I hope to see not a trace left of the
old and accursed system.

"We owe the noble position which this country occupies at the head of one great department of beneficence
and civilisation to you, Dr. Conolly, and to such as you.
I cannot confine my views merely to the physical
results of the new system. I look, also, to the moral
results, and I find that while the class of lunatics has
been raised in the moral scale of existence, society
generally has benefited. I am quite sure that all who
hear me, and all who may read these remarks, will
concur in thanking you for your great services; in
rejoicing that you have been called, and that you have
answered to the call, to do good work in your generation; and we trust that while you may long be spared
to pursue your noble and beneficent career, you may,
in the evening of your days, be made happy in the
peaceful and blessed consolation that you have been
instrumental in alleviating the miseries of mankind;
and that under the blessing of Almighty God you have
served, and effectually served, your fellow-creatures.
Allow me now, in the name of this meeting, to request
your acceptance of these testimonials as records of our
esteem, our respect, and our gratitude."

Dr. Conolly replied thus:—" It is so usual with

the recipients of public testimonials to deny their worthiness of the honour conferred on them, that it is very difficult for me to say the same thing, without exposing myself to the suspicion that I am but using the foolish language of affectation. But those who know me well, will believe me when I say there never was an occasion when the sense of merit was less reflected from the breast of the recipient of a public honour, than it is from me at this moment. Not that I wish to depreciate or undervalue the nature of the labours in which I have been engaged for so many years; nor that I wish to deny that I hope the good I have done may live after me, and lead to further good; but because I had great examples before me; that as a student I was smitten with those examples, and that my whole life has been a zealous pursuit in the path they had opened up. This occasion produces a singular effect on me. It recalls vividly all the events of my past life, my first views on the treatment of lunatics, my first ambitions in this direction, and the steps which led me to that career, now so fully and completely rewarded. My friend, Sir John Forbes, will remember that when I first heard of the establishment of Hanwell Asylum, I was seized with a restless desire to become one day the head of that establishment."

Dr. Conolly then entered upon the history of the medical treatment of the insane:—" Nothing is more extraordinary in medical history than the fact, that the Greek physicians have been imitated in the treatment of lunatics down almost to the present day. The prescriptions of Celsus, of force to subdue the ferocity and the violence of lunatics, had been followed down nearly to the end of the last century. Hoffman, the most voluminous writer among the physicians of the last century, showed what the practice throughout his time was; the patient was to be dealt with quietly when he was passive; and when he was violent, he was to be scolded and beaten with stripes. Dr. Corry, in the same period, laid it down that fear was the principle to proceed upon in treating the insane, that the readiest method of producing fear was punishment, and that the readiest punishment was stripes. Stripes, however, were but one form, and the slightest, of cruelty; in the old asylums, all the most terrible engines of torture to carry out the theory of punishment were resorted to. The inventions to give pain were marvellous. There were chairs of restraint, in which the patient could not move limb or body; and whirling chairs, in which the unfortunate lunatic was whirled round at the rate of a hundred gyrations a minute. The foreign physicians, in particular the German physicians, went even further, and contemplated tortures by forcing illusions; for instance, suggesting a means of drawing the lunatic up to the top of a high tower, and plunging him down suddenly, as he would suppose, to a deep cavern, which was to be all the better if it could be fitted with serpents; and again expatiating upon the advantage to be derived from walking a patient across a room, and making him suddenly tumble into a cistern in which he would be nearly drowned. These dreadful things had

continued until after 1790. . . . . In the asylums
the lunatics were also kept in a state of partial famine,
chained, covered with dirt and filth, but half clothed,
and those insufficient clothes seldom changed. Cages
of iron were in use, in which some of the lunatics were
kept for years and years; and all these miseries were
inflicted, not from carelessness, but from what was
believed to be real humanity. My attention was first
called to the subject by an inspection, when a youth,
of the asylum that then existed at Glasgow. About
that time I read the works of Pinel, and of Samuel
Tuke, of York, published in 1813. To those two great
and good men, society is indebted for nearly all the
improvements which followed their essays. At the
time of which I speak, the asylums in Great Britain
appeared to be competing for a bad eminence. Among
the bad, the York Asylum was the worst. In 1791,
some members of the Society of Friends sent one of
their family—a lady—for care to that asylum. The
rules of the asylum forbade her relatives to see her.
She died. Something wrong was suspected; and from
that day, the Society of Friends, acting as always in
conformity with Christian precepts, and never hesitating
to face a right because of its difficulties, determined
to establish an institution in which there should be no
secrecy. William Tuke was the great founder of the
new asylum; and from the first, he and his friends
pursued in their institution those principles which are
now universally acknowledged. Certainly restraint was
not altogether abolished by them, but they undoubt-

edly began the new system in this country; and the restraints they did continue to resort to were of the mildest kind. About the same time, a change was commencing in Paris. When the tree of liberty was shedding fast its blood-red fruit in one corner of Paris, a good and courageous man, Pinel, was acting upon a determination to liberate from their wretched prisons some lunatics who had been for years in confinement. . . . .

" In 1815, public opinion was aroused about lunatic asylums. Attention had been forced on the sad state of old Bethlehem, and there were Parliamentary Reports denouncing it, and demanding a new system. Bethlehem, with its chained rows of raging lunatics, the men on one side and the women on another side, had been a Sunday sight for the Londoners. The provincial asylums were even more frightfully conducted."

Dr. Conolly then relates some of the inhuman practices under the coercion system, and goes on to say :—

" In 1818 or 1819 new asylums were built, and the improvement commenced. I am glad to have the opportunity of testifying to the great merits of Mr. Gardner Hill, in connection with the Lincoln Asylum. Mr. Hill's claims have been somewhat injudiciously put forward, but his real claims every one has pleasure in admitting. Mr. Hill's merits have been put in contrast with my own. Now I never made any claim whatever to the merit of having been the first person to abolish restraint in asylums. In my very first Report in con-

E

nection with Hanwell, and in other publications, I
noticed how deeply I was indebted to Dr. Charlesworth,
the physician to the Lincoln Asylum, and to Mr.
Gardner Hill.   .   .   .

"In 1838 all restraint had been abolished at Lincoln,
and, perhaps, had I not seen that it was quite practicable to conduct an asylum without restraint, I might
not have had the courage to make the attempt. At
any rate, I have always and shall always acknowledge
my obligations to Dr. Charlesworth and Mr. Hill. I
went to Hanwell first in 1839. I abolished restraint
at the outset. The attendants and officers attempted
to induce me to give up my ideas, but I persevered.
I liberated all the violent at once. I never received a
blow at Hanwell, whatever my troubles elsewhere ; at
Hanwell I felt a happy man among friends.

" I never entered into controversies about the success,
or failure of, my system. My answer to all argument
was, " Come and see." After all, my system is very
simple, nothing but the exercise of a little humanity
and a little common sense, and the result explains it.
The example of Hanwell has, with time, been generally imitated; and it has been found that, with proper
regulations, what is done in the asylum can be done
with patients in a private residence. I acknowledge
heartily the aid I have received from others : from the
Middlesex magistrates, who backed me from the commencement; from the medical officers who have lived
at Hanwell, and who have passed on to the control of
other asylums, Dr. Davis, Dr. Nesbitt, and Dr. Hitch-

man ; from the medical press, and, in particular, from
Sir John Forbes and the editor of the *Lancet ;* and
lastly, from the Commissioners in Lunacy, over whom
the noble Lord in the chair has so ably and so humanely
presided. The friendship of Sir John Forbes and Sir
James Clark upheld me throughout. The honour now
conferred on me shall not make me complacent or
indolent. I hope to continue my labours for some
years, propagating the doctrines admitted to be correct,
and diffusing by communication with others the bless-
ings of the new system far and wide. In conclusion, I
humbly and sincerely thank you. I am approaching
the last arch of the mysterious bridge of life; and I
can assure you I shall go from this meeting, determined
to waste no time in enlisting the aid of the wise and
good, and so to persevere in fulfilling my duties, to
which God in His great mercy has been pleased to
call me."

V.

It must not be supposed that Dr. Conolly accomplished his work without being subjected to much obloquy and misrepresentation by the enemies of the system, of whom not a few were influenced in their enmity and opposition by interested motives; and also by others from whom he had every reason to expect moral support at least. So far, on the contrary, had this system of opposition and misrepresentation been carried, that Professor Paget, of Cambridge, in his late oration before the Royal College of Physicians, observes that "Dr. Conolly's experiment at Hanwell would have been foiled by opposition and discouragement, had he not been sustained by a spirit of earnest benevolence towards his unhappy patients."

But the difficulties and discouragements which he met with, although they may have somewhat impeded his progress, never damped Dr. Conolly's hopefulness, nor abated his energy. He felt so thoroughly impressed with the importance, and so happy in the success, of his work, that he could afford to treat the authors of the groundless attacks made upon him, with calm contempt,—aware that no great work was ever accomplished in this world without opposition and misrepresentations.

The following letter to his friend Dr. Bucknill shows the spirit in which he treated the groundless accusations to which he had been subjected, and to which Dr. Bucknill had been referring in his correspondence with Dr. Conolly. It is dated January 30, 1856.

" I have been wishing to write to you for some weeks, but occupations which in my state seem many and great, have devoured my time, or exhausted my energy, day after day. Also I am anxiously preparing the volume on *The Non-Restraint System*, which has made a reference to my diaries and manuscripts innumerable (the work of the last sixteen or seventeen years) a necessary labour,—and it has occupied much more time than I expected. These records would furnish a curious commentary on some recent attacks made on me.

"The fact is, I did not immediately succeed Sir Wm. Ellis. He resigned in 1838; and at the election, the casting vote of the Chairman (the late Colonel Clitherow) excluded me in favour of Dr. Millingen. Some time afterwards Col. C. told me that my exclusion was occasioned by my politics! In 1839, on the resignation of Dr. Millingen, I was elected by a large majority. Dr. Millingen denounced non-restraint and the system, and all the friends of the Ellises misrepresented me. Certainly I found no commencement of non-restraint in the Asylum. In every ward there was a closetful of restraints, and every attendant used them at will. Many patients were always in restraint. Six new restraint-chairs had recently been added to the stock, making forty-one. Within four months all this was done away with; but I was cruelly persecuted, and many friends of the old system were my enemies to the last. For two years Sergeant Adams was a staunch friend, and most able defender of the new system; upon which I had had repeated conferences with him immediately after my election.

" Your question has led me to say what I have said. The troubles to which I have alluded are now of no consequence. In my book I shall scarcely allude to them at all, and I shall very temperately touch on the old faults of Hanwell. I wish to view the subject as it will be viewed by others now, and in years to come. For any service that I did I have been generously repaid by public opinion, and by that of our own profession, which I chiefly value."

VI.

THE almost total neglect of insanity as a branch of medical education by our Universities and Medical Schools had long been a subject of complaint by Dr. Conolly. "The interests of the public," he remarked, " greatly require that medical men, to whom alone the insane can ever be properly trusted, should have opportunities of studying the various forms of insanity, and preparing themselves for its treatment, in the same manner in which they prepare themselves for the treatment of other disorders. They have at present no such opportunities." His opinion was, that every public lunatic asylum should be available for practical instruction. " It would be some compensation," he said, " for the unavoidable evils of public asylums, if each establishment of that kind became a clinical school, in which under certain restrictions medical students might prepare themselves for their future duties to the insane. It is true that insane patients are not always in a state to be visited by pupils, and that a very strict discipline would be necessary to prevent disorder or impropriety ; but such discipline is quite practicable, and such arrangements might be made as would at once guard those patients whom disturbance might injure, and yet present a sufficient number of instructive examples to the students."[1]

Dr. Conolly's observations are in a great degree still applicable. Insanity has not yet found a place among the *required* branches of medical education in this country. Steps, however, have been recently taken to supply in some measure this want, and no doubt insanity will soon take its proper place in the medical curriculum. The Senate of the University of London has made a small step in advance by recognising three months' attendance, with clinical instruction, in a lunatic asylum as equivalent to the same period of attendance in a medical hospital. With this view, the Senate has recognised Bethlehem and St. Luke's Hospitals as medical schools for the practical study of insanity. The lunatic asylums of Edinburgh, Glasgow, and Aberdeen, admit medical students to their wards for practical instruction, although a small number only avail themselves of the opportunity. So it will continue to be, till insanity is made a subject of examination for a medical degree.

A professor of mental diseases has been appointed by University College, London, who gives clinical instruction in an asylum, but attendance is optional. Dr. Laycock, Professor of Medicine in the University of Edinburgh, has delivered a course of lectures on Medical Psychology, and given clinical instruction in mental diseases, during the summer sessions, for the last ten years; and although the course is not recognised

[1] *Indications of Insanity.*

by the University, and is therefore voluntary, it has been attended by a considerable number of students.

When the opportunity occurred to himself, Dr. Conolly did all he could to remedy this defect in medical education, by instituting a course of clinical lectures in the Hanwell Asylum. [1]

The plan on which these lectures were arranged and conducted was admirably adapted for conveying practical instruction. One day a week was devoted to them during the summer, the early part being occupied by Dr. Conolly and the medical officers of the Asylum in conducting the advanced medical students and young physicians, who attended the lectures, through the wards, making them acquainted with the character and phases of insanity, as exhibited in the different patients, and directing their attention more especially to those cases which Dr. Conolly had selected for illustrating the afternoon lecture. No more complete course of clinical instruction on insanity was, I believe, ever given in this country; [2] and when it is considered that for six

[1] Dr. Hitchman, the present medical superintendent of the admirably conducted county asylum at Derby, was at that time one of the medical officers of the Asylum, and was of great assistance to Dr. Conolly in the preparations for these lectures.

[2] Dr. Battie, of St. Luke's Hospital, was the first in this country to give clinical instruction on insanity; and after Dr. Battie, but at a long interval, Sir Alexander Morison, when Physician to Bethlehem Hospital, gave a course of lectures on insanity from 1842 to 1852. Dr. Sutherland, Dr. Hood, and others, have also given practical lectures in St. Luke's and Bethlehem Hospitals, and Dr. W. A. F. Browne, in the Crichton Institution at Dumfries, but no systematic course of clinical lectures was, I believe, given in this country before that given by Dr. Conolly.

years the course was repeated, and was entirely gratuitous, we have a striking proof of Dr. Conolly's zeal
in promoting the practical study of insanity.

Dr. Conolly's course of clinical teaching at Hanwell
commenced in 1842, when the non-restraint system was
in full operation. "It appeared to me," he remarks,
"then only could the proper study of insanity begin;
the removal of restraints, and of all violent and irritating methods of control, thus first permitting the student
to contemplate disorders of the mind in their simplicity,
and no longer modified by exasperating treatment.
Patients could then be presented to the observation of
the students, as subjects of study and reflection."[1]

The lectures at Hanwell were impeded by many
obstacles. The assistance required in conducting them
was limited and uncertain; and after some interruptions, principally arising from this cause, Dr. Conolly
found it necessary to discontinue them.

Having learned that my friend Dr. Gull had attended
Dr. Conolly's clinical lectures at Hanwell, I asked him
to write me his opinion of them, both as regarded their
advantage to the students and their effects upon the
tranquillity of the Asylum. The following reply of Dr.
Gull is most satisfactory on both points :—

"I regret your note should have remained so long
unanswered, but I have not had a convenient time to
reply to it, and I was unwilling to answer it cursorily.

"I had the advantage of attending the clinical lectures
given by Dr. Conolly at the Hanwell Asylum; and I

[1] *Treatment of the Insane*, pp. 298, 299.

retain the most vivid and pleasant remembrance of
them. Two students were nominated from each of the
metropolitan hospitals to form this clinical class. We
assembled at Hanwell about noon once a week. We
then made a visit through the wards in company with
Dr. Conolly and the medical officers of the Asylum,
receiving some words of instruction upon the cases in
general, our attention being especially directed to
particular patients. This occupied, probably, near
two hours; I believe sometimes more. We thus,
from week to week, saw almost every phase of mental
disorder, from acute mania to general paralysis and
dementia. We also saw the application of the system of
non-restraint, then on its trial, directed by that kind and
calm philosophic temper so very conspicuous in Dr.
Conolly. I cannot express to you the charm we all felt
in these visits. The Asylum in the country, apart from
the noise and bustle of the town; the novelty of the
clinical work and teaching ; the new field of facts before
us, contrasting with those afforded in the routine of our
other hospitals ; the feeling of the peculiar advantages
thus enjoyed—all combined to make us eager and
thankful. I have often regretted that such great opportunities have been since neglected, and that year by
year these large fields of knowledge have been lying
waste and barren. If by any word you could awaken
again the minds of those who govern and direct these
institutions, so that they might make them available for
medical instruction, after the manner inaugurated by
Dr. Conolly, you would indeed prove a benefactor to us

all. It is lamentable to think what ignorance yet prevails in and out of our profession on the subject of insanity. So it will be, whilst the matter remains a special study. The prejudice was too strong for even Dr. Conolly. He set a bright example, but the difficulties were too great for him. I should, indeed, be glad to think that others should in long succession enjoy such opportunities as we had at Hanwell.

"I can also satisfactorily answer your inquiry respecting the effect of our visits upon the inmates of the Asylum. To the great majority it was a matter of indifference, or of some interest, and to others it seemed to give pleasure. Generally the visits round the wards was with as little inconvenience to the patients as it would have been had it been in the wards of a hospital for general diseases. There were occasions when it was necessary to caution the students against approaching or addressing certain cases, when, from some mental peculiarity, any familiarity would have caused excitement. As such cases were known beforehand to the physician, they were easily avoided, whilst they, at the same time, afforded important clinical hints. I may here say that this course of instruction in the Asylum necessitated and enforced a careful demeanour of the students.

"The cases of acute mania requiring entire quiet and seclusion are rare in all asylums, but even these could often be seen unobserved through the wickets of the padded rooms in which they were confined, without disturbance, whilst the physician supplied the closer facts of each case, and directed our minds to the proper consideration of them. When the severity of the attack was passing off, Dr. Conolly would, at his discretion, permit us to have a closer study of such cases, in the same way that in our general hospitals the severer diseases are guarded by the physician against injurious examinations. In all the visits I paid to Hanwell, I never saw anything caused by the presence of the students, which militated against the good order of the establishment or the welfare of the patients.

"From what I saw at Hanwell, and from my experience since, I have no doubt of the practicability of making the public lunatic asylums schools for medical men and jurists, without detriment to the inmates. On the contrary, if this were done, much good must accrue every way. Nothing develops those establishments so much as making them centres of scientific observation and practical instruction. Without this our large hospitals would have been but infirmaries, and the sick would certainly not have had the best treatment.

"The debt I owe to Dr. Conolly obliges me to incur the risk of being tedious, if thereby I may express my obligations to his memory.

"*Dec.* 25, 1866."

Of the excellence of Dr. Conolly's clinical lectures, the reasoned opinion of Dr. Gull is conclusive, and I now know that it is in accordance with that of other physicians, well qualified to judge, who also attended

these lectures and who look back on Conolly's teaching
with the same feelings as Dr. Gull, both as to their
great practical usefulness, and the facility with which
such clinical lessons may be conducted in every well-
managed asylum where non-restraint is practised, without injury or inconvenience to the patients, and with
great advantage to the profession and the public.

It is to be hoped that the time is not far distant
when every graduate, before obtaining a license to
practise medicine, shall be required to have attended
such a clinical course, and to have given special evidence of his knowledge of the subject. Of the necessity
of a knowledge of mental diseases no practical physician
entertains the smallest doubt. Sir Henry Holland
justly remarks, " Scarcely can we name a morbid
affection of the body in which some feeling or function
of the mind is not concurrently engaged, directly or
indirectly, as cause or effect.[1]

The subjects of medical instruction which are left
optional, of which Insanity is one, are neglected by the
majority of students. The authorities of the medical
schools are aware of this, but they feel reluctant to
increase the requirements of the student beyond what
he can accomplish in the time allotted to his professional education. The truth is, medical science has
made such progress, and the subjects embraced by it
are so much extended within the present century, that
the former medical curriculum is totally inadequate to
enable the student of the present day to acquire a com-

---

[1] *Chapters on Mental Physiology*—Preface.

petent knowledge of the numerous subjects required of him, before he can obtain a medical degree.

The Senate of the University of London, from the date of its establishment, directed its attention to the improvement of medical education, and especially to the finding of a remedy for the then defective state of the preliminary instruction in literature and science, requisite to prepare the student for entering with advantage on his medical studies; and in this they have succeeded by their regulations, and by the effects of their example on the medical schools and licensing bodies throughout the kingdom, to an extent which those only are capable of estimating, who know the state of medical education when the University was founded in 1838. One of the recent and most important steps made by the Senate in this direction was to constitute a *scientific examination* between *matriculation* and the commencement of the proper *medical curriculum.* A knowledge of the subjects required by this regulation is of the utmost advantage to the student. The acquirement of it habituates his mind to close observation and methodical habits of study, and thus forms an excellent preparation for entering on his course of professional instruction. But notwithstanding the advantage afforded by these preparatory studies in facilitating and lightening the labours of the strictly professional education, the present medical curriculum of four years is clearly insufficient to enable the majority of students to acquire a proper knowledge of their profession, and it would be well that the parents of youths designed for the medical profession, should be made aware of this.

THE CLINICAL TEACHING OF INSANITY has made much less progress in asylums than might justly have been looked for. The credit of the first attempt to instruct students by actual observation of the phenomena of madness, belongs to St. Luke's Hospital under the auspices of its first physician (in 1750), Dr. Battie. But the excellent example thus set has been singularly unproductive of imitators in England, which at the present day affords the most scanty opportunities to medical men to study the pathology and treatment of mental disorders ; and indeed offers no adequate inducement to them to undertake the study by making it an integral portion of the medical curriculum.

In France likewise, the pursuit of psychological medicine does not obtain its proper recognition in the course of medical education. Time occupied in the study of that subject is, however, allowed to count in the career of the student, and by the system of "internes," each asylum happily is rendered available for practical instruction. Clinical lectures, moreover, have been delivered in Paris since the time of Esquirol.

In Germany more definite and persevering attempts at clinical teaching have been continued since 1817, when Horn commenced a course of lectures at Berlin. In Leipzig, Wurzburg and Sonnenstein, Horn's example was at once followed ; and at the present day, theoretical in some, and practical instruction in insanity in

other university towns, is given, though not, we believe,
made essential in the programmes of the examining
boards.

In Italy, a chair of mental pathology was first instituted in Florence in 1840. The example was followed
in Turin in 1850, in Bologna in 1860, and in Naples in
1863. In the last named city, the energetic physician
of Aversa, Miraglia, is the professor and practical
instructor. Recently, lectures were delivered in six of
the Italian universities, and what is of more importance,
is, as Dr. Bacon informs us, that every student for
a medical degree, has to produce evidence of having
attended clinically the study of mental disorders.

VII.

IN his clinical lectures, and on other occasions, Dr. Conolly was in the habit of pointing out the assistance afforded by phrenology in the diagnosis and treatment of lunacy. In his *Indications of Insanity*, for instance, when commenting on a case in which the perceptive faculties and physical energy were active, while the reflective faculties had not sufficient controlling power, he expresses his opinion in the following terms :—

" This is not the only variety of character of which it may occur to some of my readers, that the phrenological system affords the best apparent explanation. The facts alluded to in the text, many of the phenomena of disease, and the observation of all mankind, seem to me to prove that the first principles of phrenology are founded in nature. On these it is very probable that many fancies and errors may have been built; but now that anatomy and physiology have together penetrated so far into the separateness of the structure and functions of the nerves of the spinal marrow, and even of certain portions of the cerebral mass, I can see nothing which merits the praise of being philosophical, in the real or affected contempt professed by so many anatomists and physiologists, for a science which, however imperfect, has for its object the demonstration that, for other functions the existence of which none can deny, there are further separations and distinctions of hitherto unexplained portions of nervous matter." [1]

At a later period, in one of the Lectures on Mental Disease, which he delivered in the Royal Institution, he gave the following rational view of phrenology :—

"Although the doctrines of phrenology have met with little favour, and the pretensions of recent professors of occult methods of acting upon the nervous system, have thrown an air of absurdity even over the truths of what is called phrenology, no person not altogether devoid of the power of observation can affect to overlook the general importance of the shape and even of the size of the brain in relation to the development of the mental faculties. It is reasonable to consider each of the large and marked divisions of the brain, and each of the convolutions, with their copious supply of grey or vesicular nerve-substance, as possessing distinct offices; and the more or less perfect development of these several masses, and the greater or less nervous energy they possess, as circumstances connected with the varieties of mental character, and with the disordered manifestations of the mind. Each mass, or each subdivision of such mass, may, like each nerve, have a distinct office. Each, however, excited, may only be capable of one kind of manifestation of the excitement. Each, when in a healthy state, may be excited

---

[1] *Indications of Insanity*, p. 135.

F 2

simultaneously throughout; and each in disease may
be excited irregularly, or too long, or lose the power of
being excited altogether."

Again, in the subjoined extract from a letter to the
late George Combe, he thus expresses his belief in
the value of a regard to the principles of phrenology
in the treatment of mental diseases :—

" Many and pressing avocations leave me no time
just at present to express to you, in a manner at all
worthy of the subject, my conviction of the great usefulness of habitual regard to the principles of phrenology, especially in my department of practice, and of
the confusion and imperfection of the views which seem
to me to be taken, both of sound and unsound mind,
by those who reject the aid of observations confirmed
now by vast experience, and most of which may be
daily verified in asylums for the insane. I am also
convinced, that attention to the form of the head, con-
joined with that cautious consideration of all other
physical circumstances which no prudent phrenologist
disregards, will often enable the practitioner to form
an accurate prognosis in cases of mental disorder, and
to foretel the chances of recovery or amelioration, or
hopeless and gradual deterioration."

In his work on *Mental Derangement*, Dr. Andrew
Combe expresses his opinion on the value of phrenology in the treatment of insanity in still more decided
terms. "Ignorance of the philosophy of the human
mind," he says, " and of its relations to the brain as
its material organ, is one of the greatest obstacles,

not only to the present cure of the insane, but to
the farther advancement of our medical knowledge of
insanity; and till this truth shall be recognised in
its fullest force, and the principles of phrenology be
adopted as the physiological, and therefore the surest,
basis of a mental philosophy, we shall look in vain for
those ameliorations in the management of the insane
which are so imperatively required." [1]

Dr. Combe's work just referred to, independently of
phrenological doctrines, may, for its sound sense and
the rational principles which it inculcates on Insanity,
more especially as regards its prevention, be placed
fairly beside Conolly's ' Indications,' as a work that
should be carefully read by every student of mental
disease.

Sir Henry Holland, although no phrenologist, admits
that " the phrenologists rightly regard it as probable,
or even as proved, that there is a certain plurality of
parts in the total structure of the brain, corresponding
to, and having connexion with, the different intellectual
and moral faculties. The undoubted natural diversity
of these faculties makes this probable, seeing that we
must regard a certain organization as ministering in
the present life even to the higher powers of our nature.
The partial and varying effects of accident, disease, or
other less obvious change in the brain, in producing
derangement of the mental functions, furnish more

---

[1] *Observations on Mental Derangement: being an application of
the Principles of Phrenology to the elucidation of the causes, symptoms, nature, and treatment of Insanity*, p. 350.   Edinb., 1831.

direct evidence, and such as we cannot refuse to admit." [1]

Cuvier, again, expresses his opinion in the following equally strong terms. As " certain parts of the brain," he says, " attain, in all classes of animals, a development proportioned to the peculiar properties of these animals, one may hope, by following up these researches, at length to acquire some notion of the particular uses of each part of the brain." [2]

" Phrenology in its present state," as Dr. Conolly remarks, " may be held in small estimation, yet there are not wanting grounds for the belief, that its leading principles rest on truth, and that ultimately its value may receive a general acknowledgment. It seems reasonable, indeed, to *expect* the brain to be an aggregate of different parts, each subserving the manifestation of a particular mental function. Such a view has assuredly the support of analogy, being quite consistent with our knowledge of the manner in which other organs discharge complicated functions, and it also derives direct support from researches, both recent and old, into the anatomy and physiology of the brain itself."

Professor Turner, in his late description of the convolutions of the human brain, makes the following statements:—

" Our knowledge not only of the form, size, and relations of the great subdivisions of the hemisphere,

---

[1] *Chapters on Mental Physiology*, p. 192.
[2] *British and Foreign Medical Review*, vol. ix. p. 200.

but of the topography of the individual convolutions, has been very materially advanced; so much so, indeed, that we can now localize the different . gyri, and give to each its appropriate name."[1] And towards the conclusion of his paper, he says further: "The precise morphological investigations of the last few years into the cerebral convolutions have led to the revival in Paris of discussions, in which the doctrine of Gall and his disciples—that the brain is not one but consists of many organs — has been supported by new arguments, and the opinion has been expressed that the primary convolutions, at least, are both morphologically and physiologically distinct organs."[2]

Recent discoveries in the researches of other men have led them to express similar thoughts, and sometimes in a way which cannot fail to attract the attention both of physiologists and physicians.   Dr. Richardson, for example, a gentleman of distinction in scientific inquiry, in one of his late lectures on *Experimental and Practical Medicine*,[3] thus gives the reflections, which are suggested to him by the results of his own and other recent investigations.

"It appears to us," he says, "as though the brain were not made up of portions of the same matter all united into one organism, but as though it were dis-

[1] *The Convolutions of the Human Cerebrum Topographically Considered*, by William Turner, M.B., Professor of Anatomy in the University of Edinburgh, 1866.

[2] *Op. cit.* p. 27.

[3] *Medical Times Gazette*, 1867.

tinctly mapped out into insular divisions, each well separated from its neighbour, and having its own duties.

.   .   .   .   .   .

"In describing this local independency of nervous function, I refer of course specially to physical facts, not to those metaphysical, or I had better have said psychological, arguments which the illustrious Gall instituted in regard to the isolation and development of the organs of the mind."

These observations, which are founded on inquiries into the anatomy and physiology of the brain, strengthened by recent discoveries in pathology, all point in one direction, and tend to support the opinion of phrenologists that the brain is an aggregate of many different parts, each appropriated to the manifestation of a particular mental faculty. The prediction, therefore, of the late Dr. Andrew Combe, the most sagacious and far-seeing of all British writers on Phrenology, that a possible position of importance awaited it in the future, appears to rest on a surer foundation than has been sometimes imagined :—"If phrenology is true," says Dr. Combe, and we know that he firmly believed in its truth, "it furnishes a key, not only to the physiology of the brain and nervous system, but to the philosophy of the mind."[1]

---

[1] *Address on Phrenology, its Nature and Uses,* p. 12.   Edinburgh, 1846.

VIII.

DR. CONOLLY was strongly impressed with the importance of a well-directed system of education as a means of developing and strengthening the mental faculties in girls; and his remarks on insanity, having its remote origin in imperfect or mis-directed education, are so important that I have thought them deserving of particular notice. After referring to the provision now made for the " education and training of those children in whom imbecility is clearly recognized,—a special training conducted in their case, on principles which are in strict accordance with the dictates of science,"— he observes that in the education of children generally, " nothing is so conspicuous as a steady disregard of physiological principles," and he then proceeds to speak thus of what has been observed in asylums to be often true of the education of their inmates. " All who have peculiar opportunities of ascertaining the mental habits of insane persons of the educated classes, well know that, with some exceptions, their previous studies and pursuits appear to have been superficial and desultory, and often frivolous. The condition of the female mind is, even in the highest classes, too often more deplorable still. Not only is it most rare to find them

familiar with the best authors of their own country,
but most common to find that they have never read a
really good author either in their own or in any other
language ; and that the few accomplishments possessed
by them have been taught for display in society, and
not for solace in quieter hours.   All this has been said
before and often, but in vain."   He further adds, "there
is a frequent perversion of intellectual exercise, more
fatal than its omission, which fills asylums with lady
patients terrified by metaphysical translations, and be-
wildered by religious romances, and who have lost all
custom of healthful exercise of body and mind,—all love
of natural objects—all interest in things most largely
influencing the happiness of mankind.   These evils
have generally taken deep root before the patient's
manifest want of reasonable constraint induces a resort
to an asylum."

The importance of Dr. Conolly's views on the de-
moralizing effects on the minds of young females of
misdirected education, which is so general, deserves the
serious consideration of parents.[1]   What adds to the
importance of a well-directed education in the case of
girls, more especially of those belonging to families
where an hereditary taint is known to exist, is the fact
that the tendency to insanity is believed to be more
frequently transmitted to the offspring by the mother
than by the father.

The present movement to improve and elevate the

---

[1] *On the Treatment of the Insane,* p. 160, &c.

character of female education, cannot fail to act bene-
ficially as a means of developing and strengthening the
mind, and of storing it with such sound and useful
knowledge as will fit the sex for those important duties
in life which are clearly indicated by the Creator as
suited to the nature of the female constitution, both
mental and physical.

IX.

AFTER giving the history of the progress of non-restraint
in Hanwell Asylum, Dr. Conolly speaks of its ready
adoption by the medical superintendents of our county
asylums in the following gratifying words :—" As soon
as the new system of treatment had been fairly tried at
Hanwell it began to be adopted by the superintendents
of several English asylums approaching nearest to
Hanwell in size. Success followed everywhere. It was
invariably found that when there was a determination
to manage all cases of insanity without resorting to the
employment of mechanical coercion, it was practicable
and safe, and advantageous to do so." [1]

This ready acceptance of the non-restraint system
introduced into Hanwell Asylum by Dr. Conolly, is
highly creditable to the intelligence and benevolent
feelings of the medical superintendents of asylums.
That a treatment differing so widely from that which
had hitherto been in universal practice, with the single
exception of the small asylum of Lincoln, should be so
speedily and generally adopted, was contrary to the
experience of what usually happens in the progress of
such a radical change in a long established practice ;

---

[1] *Treatment of the Insane,* p. 290.

and the more so as the change in this case entailed a great increase in the labour, the vigilance, and anxiety of the superintendents of asylums.

The following extracts from some of the asylum Reports, showing the state of our asylums before the introduction of non-restraint, and after time had been allowed to show its effects, cannot fail to be read with interest.

Dr. Conolly mentions several of the medical superintendents of asylums who were among the earliest to follow the example of Hanwell. He refers especially to Mr. Gaskell, now a retired Commissioner in Lunacy, then Medical Superintendent of the Lancaster Asylum, as one of the first to adopt the *non-restraint system*, which, Dr. Conolly remarks, " he carried out with singular ability and success in an asylum containing 600 patients, considered to be of a proverbially rough character."

The following is an extract from the Report for 1855 of the County Asylum of Lancaster, by Dr. Vitre, the Visiting Physician, and Mr. Broadhurst, the Medical Superintendent. Mr. Gaskell, with whom the reforms in this asylum originated, was succeeded by Mr. Broadhurst, who has ably continued what his friend began :—

" Previous to the year 1840, mechanical restraint formed the *rule* of practice rather than the exception ; all cases on admission were at night placed under restraint, and were only released when, from familiarity

with their symptoms, it was thought they could be
trusted without.   Two large compartments in the
Asylum were fitted up with a variety of mechanical
contrivances for the constant restraint of refractory
patients.   These compartments contained a row of
stalled seats, surrounding nearly two-thirds of the wall
in each room, and served the double purpose of a
water-closet and an ordinary seat; the flagged floors
were heated by hot air, and the patients were secured
by hand-locks to each side of the upper portion of the
stalls, and by leg-locks to the lower portion, the heated
floor superseding the necessity of stockings and shoes;
all the bedsteads, and many of the fixed seats were so
constructed as readily to admit of the free use of mechanical means to restrain their occupants.

"Early in the spring of 1840 an attempt was made
by Mr. Gaskell to mitigate the horrors of such a mode
of treatment; and with the cordial sanction and appro-
bation of the Visiting Magistrates, these compartments
were speedily abolished, along with all other forms of
mechanical restraint then in common use in all parts
of the establishment.   Since the above period, upwards
of 3000 patients have been under treatment, and only
in *one instance* has it been deemed necessary to have
recourse to mechanical restraint.

"An appeal can now be confidently made to the
statistics of the Asylum, in proof of the unspeakable
advantages of moral over mechanical means of treatment, as observable in the general *quietness* and de-
corum of the establishment, in the cheerful aspect of

the patients, in the comparative freedom from acts
of destructive violence, and in the large proportion of
inmates who are constantly engaged in some useful
occupation; to which might be added, a *decreased mortality*, and an *increased percentage* of *cures*."

Mr. Wilkes, now one of the Commissioners in
Lunacy, then Medical Superintendent of the Stafford
County Asylum, writes thus in 1855 of the effects
of liberating the insane from mechanical restraint:—
" The effect of this change upon the old inmates of
the Asylum was in a marked degree beneficial; one
patient who had been regarded as incurable and for
a length of time had been wearing the muff and
hobbles, rapidly improved upon being set at liberty,
and ultimately recovered. The excitement of the
patients generally was decidedly diminished; they were
less noisy and restless at night, and destructive propensities and objectionable habits were, in many instances,
gradually overcome. With greater opportunities of
doing mischief, less absolutely occurred; and now, without a window in the Asylum in any way protected, and
with a much larger number of patients, there is probably less breakage of glass than ever there was. . . .
The evil of the system of restraint was not simply
confined to the coercion of the patients, but the principle pervaded the whole establishment. Above all,
it was evident that the system had a tendency to
demoralize, if not to brutalize the attendants, and one
of the most important results of the disuse of restraint

is the marked effect it has had upon the feelings and
conduct of the attendants themselves."

Dr. Loyd Williams and Mr. Jones of the North Wales
Asylum, express their opinion of restraint thus (1855):—
" We have no hesitation in saying, that we have hitherto
never had occasion to resort to anything beyond a short
confinement in a padded room, and even that remedy
is now very sparingly and cautiously used. We find
exercise in the open air the best sedative, in promoting
sleep and tranquillity even during the most violent
maniacal paroxysms."

These extracts might have been largely increased,
but sufficient has been given to show the condition of
our asylums before *non-restraint* was adopted, and the
beneficial effects which its adoption produced on both
patients and attendants.

Dr. Conolly, however, thus refers to another careful
observer, the late Dr. Anderson, who visited Hanwell
several times on his appointment as Superintendent of
the Lunatic Asylum attached to the Royal Naval
Hospital at Haslar :—
"Previous to his taking the charge of the patients
there, then about one hundred and twenty in number,
including twenty or thirty naval officers, some of the
patients were constantly in restraints, being accounted
incurably dangerous. One of them was always in handcuffs ; but he had learned to put his hands into all of

his several pockets, and to use them so freely that
the protection was merely imaginary, and the restraint merely unnecessarily troublesome and vexatious.
Eighteen patients slept in iron handcuffs chained to
their beds ; their feet also being fastened. There were,
however, no restraint-chairs in the building. To all the
windows there were heavy iron bars. The patients were
not entrusted with knives and forks. In the airing-
courts there were many refreshing plots of grass, but
the patients were not allowed to walk on them. There
were no shrubberies. The view of the sea, of Portsmouth
Harbour, and of the Isle of Wight, was shut out by
very high walls. Dr. Anderson had not been long there
before everything underwent a favourable change.
Restraints were entirely abolished; iron bars disap-
peared ; the boundary walls were lowered ; the patients
were allowed to walk upon the grass; summer-houses
were built, and pleasant seats provided commanding a
view of the sea, and the cheerful scenes most congenial
to the inmates ; knives and forks were brought into use—
and the whole of this noble asylum assumed an air of
tranquil comfort. The patients soon had a large boat
provided for them, in which their good physician did
not hesitate to trust himself with parties of them in
fishing excursions. In the first of these little voyages
a patient, whose voice had not been heard for years,
was so delighted with his success that he counted his
fish aloud. These changes were all effected without
accident or inconvenience. The patients reputed to be
dangerous had, under this new management, proved to

G

be trustworthy, and some of them became industriously occupied." [1]

Dr. Bryson, the present Medical Director-General of the Navy, informs me that the Naval Asylum conducted on the non-restraint system, including the boating excursions introduced by Dr. Anderson, has been carried on without the occurrence of a single accident. The Asylum is now separated from the Naval Hospital, but is still on the coast. It contains 34 officers and 150 seamen and marines, under the superintendence of Dr. Macleod, Deputy Inspector of Hospitals, aided by a naval staff surgeon. A letter from Dr. Macleod dated January, 1869, describes the Asylum as in all respects in an excellent state. No object of mechanical restraint exists in the hospital. There is a padded room, but it is seldom used; and during the last eight months of 1868 there had not been one patient in seclusion. Nothing, indeed, can be more satisfactory than Dr. Macleod's description of the whole management of this Asylum.

In order to bring up the history of non-restraint to the present time, I requested through the Earl of Shaftesbury, Chairman of the Commission in Lunacy, to be informed as to the present treatment adopted in our public asylums, both public and private, in England and Wales, and I have been favoured by Mr. Wilkes, one of the Commissioners in Lunacy for England, with the following statement:—

---

[1] *Treatment of Insanity*, p. 296.

"It will be seen upon reference to the 'Further Report of the Commissioners in Lunacy,' published in 1847, that the use of mechanical restraint was at that period greatly diminished, and seldom or never resorted to in the best conducted county asylums. In licensed houses also its employment had been, in a great measure, laid aside, though in some, especially those receiving paupers, it was thought impracticable to avoid its occasional use without incurring the risk of serious accidents.

"The following remarks will be found at page 238 of this Report:—'A strong impression was made on the feelings and opinion of the public in reference to the treatment of lunatics, by the publication of Mr. Tuke's account of the Retreat at York. The able writings of Dr. Conolly have of late years contributed greatly to strengthen that impression, and to bring about a much more humane treatment of lunatics in many provincial asylums than that which formerly prevailed. But the Report of the Metropolitan Commissioners of 1844 affords proof that this amelioration had not extended itself to all establishments for the insane, and that much severe and needless restraint continued to be practised in numerous private and in some public asylums.'

"The opinions of the various medical superintendents and proprietors of county and borough asylums, registered hospitals, and licensed houses, on the subject of the employment of mechanical restraint in the treatment of the insane, will be found in the Commissioners' 8th Report, published in 1854, and at page 42 the following paragraph occurs:—' As a general result which may fairly be deduced from a careful examination and review of the whole body of information thus collected, we feel ourselves fully warranted in stating that the disuse of instrumental restraint, as unnecessary and injurious to the patients, is practically the rule in nearly all the public institutions in the kingdom, and generally also in the best conducted private asylums, even those where the 'non-restraint system,' as an abstract principle, admitting of no deviation or exception, has not in terms been adopted.'

" Subsequent years have witnessed the further gradual disuse of restraint in the treatment of the insane in this country, but still exceptional cases occur from time to time both in public and private asylums, in which its employment is considered desirable.

" In many of these cases it is used exclusively for surgical reasons, usually to prevent patients removing dressings from, or interfering with, wounds or injuries they may have received ; in others in consequence of inveterate tendencies to suicide or self-mutilation ; and, again, in others for acts of violence or destructiveness.   In most of these restraint is used only during the night.

" From the Reports made by the Visiting Commissioners during the past year of visits to the 66 public asylums in England and Wales, containing on the 1st January last an aggregate of 27,436 patients, it will be seen that restraint is noticed as having been employed in eleven of them, and applicable to 47 patients.   In 14 of these cases it was only used on one occasion, and in a large number of the instances it appears to have been employed for surgical reasons alone.

" At one period restraint was rather freely employed in the North Riding Asylum, near York; but since the appointment of the present Medical Superintendent it has been entirely abolished, and in no asylum can it now be said to be systematically adopted.

" The records of visits made to the various licensed houses during 1866 show that out of the 41 in the metropolitan district containing on the 1st of January last 2493 patients, restraint had been used in eight of them, and in the cases of nine of the inmates. Out of the 63 provincial licensed houses, containing 1985 patients, records of the employment of restraint had been met with in 21 of them, and applicable to 49 patients. In many of these instances, both in the metropolitan and provincial houses, it had only been used on one occasion, and for very brief periods, and was frequently employed for surgical reasons alone, and during the night.

" In many of the English asylums, both public and private, restraint is never employed ; and the cases specified above, in which it is found to be resorted to, are, in the majority of instances, of so peculiar a character, and it is used for such short periods, that such exceptions to a practice generally prevailing cannot be said to constitute any material departure from the principle of non-restraint, which is the distinguishing mark of the present treatment of insanity in England."

For the subjoined account of the present system of treatment in the Scotch asylums I am indebted to my friend Sir James Coxe, Commissioner in Lunacy for Scotland :—

"In none of the public or district asylums of Scotland is recourse ever had to mechanical restraint except on rare and special occasions, and generally for surgical reasons; for instance, to prevent the removal of dressings, or to limit motion where a bone has been fractured. Occasionally, however, the use of canvas or stiff leather gloves is sanctioned, to prevent the removal or destruction of clothing; but in a circuit embracing all the asylums in Scotland, only three or four such cases may be found.

" Non-restraint had already become the rule when the Scotch Commission of Inquiry was nominated in 1855 : but an almost equal evil had taken its place. Patients were locked up in darkened rooms for days, weeks, and even months, and not unfrequently in nakedness and filth. The rooms were cleansed perhaps only once a day, and often very imperfectly; now, such a state of matters is never seen. Indeed, in some asylums, as that of Montrose, seclusion is virtually abolished, and no one is kept in solitude except for medical reasons. Locking-up for simple excitement or refractory behaviour is repudiated. In other asylums, such as those of Edinburgh and Glasgow, in each of which it was formerly not unusual to find from four to six patients in seclusion, perhaps not one may be now so found, or only one or two, and then always in cleanliness and decency.

I have not seen a patient kept in nakedness for many
years. Much of this satisfactory state of matters is no
doubt due to the zeal and intelligence of the Medical
Superintendents; but I look upon the practice of pub-
lishing *in extenso*, adopted by the Scotch Board, of
whatever the Commissioners report at their inspections,
as being of essential service in checking abuses."

These two valuable documents afford ample proof of
the greatly improved, I may say excellent, condition of
our pauper lunatic asylums, and I have the satisfaction of adding the opinion of a gentleman well acquainted with the state of foreign lunatic asylums, as
well as those in this country, that "in no country in
the world are the asylums for the insane so well conducted as in Great Britain."

Professor Paget, of Cambridge University, in his late
elegant Harveian oration, pays the following just
compliment to our asylums:—"To my eyes, a pauper
lunatic asylum, such as may now be seen in our
English counties, with its pleasant grounds, its airy
and cleanly wards, its many comforts, and wise and
kindly superintendence, provided for those whose lot it
is to bear the double burden of poverty and mental
derangement—I say this sight is to me the most
blessed manifestation of true civilisation that the world
can present. This we owe to the courage and philanthropy of such men as Pinel and Conolly."[1]

[1] *Harveian Oration*, 1866, p. 34.

X.

ALTHOUGH we have reason to congratulate ourselves on the condition of our establishments for the care and treatment of the insane, there still remains ample room for improvement. The medical attendance in many of our asylums is inadequate,—the size of not a few of them is being increased to an extent which threatens to render them totally unsuited to the proper treatment of the insane, and not even well suited for the purpose of receptacles for chronic and incurable cases.

The number of medical officers in our public asylums bears no sound relation in general to the number of patients, more especially where the proportion of recent and curable cases is considerable. The professional duties of the medical superintendents are also in many of our county asylums too much interfered with by the performance of duties, connected with the economy of the institution, which might be better allotted to an officer appointed for such purposes; thus leaving the physician free to devote his time and attention to the treatment of the patients, and the sanitary arrangements of the institution, over which, and over every officer and individual within its walls, the medical superintendent ought to have entire control. The present state of things has a serious effect on the scientific character and usefulness of our asylums. "If," says Dr. Conolly, "the public would really estimate the consequences of the present inadequate number of medical officers in relation to the duties, which at least ought to be performed in asylums, an augmentation would be insisted upon. With the various interruptions to which they are liable, it is quite evident that two medical officers cannot sufficiently superintend a thousand patients; that they cannot even visit the wards sufficiently often without exhaustion, and consequently cannot exercise due supervision over the attendants; that on numerous occasions important duties must be omitted, and important circumstances overlooked; and that many special moral appliances must be neglected, with serious consequences to the patients, not the less real because they are unrecorded.

Without a very efficient superintendence, chiefly to be exercised by the medical officers, or rather by a chief medical officer, the mere absence of mechanical restraint may constitute no sufficient security against the neglect or even the actual ill-treatment of insane persons in a large asylum. The medical officers of asylums who consider such watchful superintendence not properly comprised in their duties have formed a very inadequate conception of them."

The excessive duties imposed on the medical officers of our asylums are strongly commented upon by foreign physicians who have visited this country. M. Morel, an eminent French alienist physician, after remarking on the amount of the duties required of our medical superintendents, and the zeal with which they are performed, adds — " mais je ne crains pas de dire qu'ils succombent à une tâche au-dessus de leurs forces." One important consequence of such excessive, and sometimes scarcely professional, duties imposed on the medical officers of our asylums, is the want of time for that close observation of their patients which is requisite to enable them to make use of the means afforded by every asylum of increasing our knowledge of the nature and treatment of mental diseases.   In this respect M. Morel compares, very unfavourably, our asylum organization and usefulness to that of France.   " Je suis fondé à croire," he writes, " que tout ce qui tient au traitement médical proprement dit, à l'observation scientifique des malades, ainsi qu'à la conservation des bonnes traditions médicales dans un asile, reçoit en notre pays une impulsion plus large." [1]

This ought not to be; it is unjust to the patients, and injurious to the character of the medical superintendents and to the usefulness of our asylums.

The increasing size of our asylums was strongly objected to by Dr. Conolly, as injurious in every respect to the comfort and treatment of the insane, and he frequently expressed his opinion on the subject in strong terms, both in conversation and in correspondence.   In a letter to the author of this memoir in 1859 he

[1] *Le Non-Restraint dans le Traitement de la Folie*, p. 26.

remarks,—" In the monstrous asylums of Hanwell and Colney Hatch, sanitary principles have been forgotten, and efficient superintendence is impossible. The magistrates go on adding wing to wing, and storey to storey, contrary to the opinion of the profession and to common sense, rendering the institution most unfavourable to the treatment of the patients, and their management most harassing and unsatisfactory to the medical superintendents." Dr. Arlidge condemns in equally strong terms the evil consequences resulting from such overgrown asylums—" Such aggregations as of 1000 to 2000 insane persons are unwieldy and unmanageable with the best appointed medical staff, unless this be so numerous as utterly to invalidate the plea of economy, the only one, fallacious as it is, that can be adduced by the advocates for their existence. And not only are they unmanageable, but also hygienically wrong; for it is a well recognised fact that the accumulation of large numbers of human beings in one place tends to engender endemic disease, uniformly deteriorates the health, and favours the onset, progress, and fatality of all disorders." [1]

The inspection of our public and private asylums is admirably conducted, but it certainly is not more than is requisite. Over the insane in private dwellings, particularly over pauper patients, of whom there are upwards of six thousand in England and Wales, there cannot be

[1] *On the State of Lunacy, &c., with Observations on the Construction and Organization of Asylums.* London, Churchill, 1859, p. 119.

said to be any direct supervision on the part of the State, no machinery for that purpose existing. Since the Commission in Lunacy was first instituted in 1843, the number of pauper lunatics in asylums has increased from 10,801 in 1849 to 25,998 in 1867, while the number of Commissioners has remained the same. Their work, therefore, which has been productive of extraordinary benefits to the insane poor of this country, and indirectly to the insane poor of other countries, must now prove very laborious.

The point, however, which presses most urgently on the consideration of the magistrates and others who have the management of our pauper asylums, is their crowded state, which seems increasing year by year. In England and Wales the annual increase has been for some time about a thousand; last year it was one thousand four hundred. The overcrowded state of our asylums is attended with several serious evils; one of the greatest of these is that it prevents the ready admission of recent cases at a time when they are most likely to be cured, and in judging of this evil it must be remembered that a large proportion of the actual inmates of our asylums consists of the incurable, of whom many are said to be harmless.

There can be little doubt that the aggregation of the insane in large numbers in asylums has been greatly fostered by the requirements and exigencies of modern social life. A lunatic is now more in the way, interferes more with business and pleasure, than was the case in ruder states of society, and his removal from the family circle is accordingly more generally desired. It cannot, however, be denied that special treatment is required in a large number of cases, and that this treatment can only be provided in establishments with special appliances. But the admission of this fact should not be allowed to interfere with the recognition of another equally important, namely, that for the efficient care and treatment of even a larger proportion of the insane, nothing is required beyond what is dictated by the general rules of good sense and benevolence.

The constant pressure for extending the existing asylum accommodation is felt almost exclusively for pauper patients. Thus, while in England the number of the private insane remains nearly stationary, that of the pauper insane has for a considerable period shown a steady increase of about a thousand a year. The principal cause of this difference is to be found in the much larger proportion of private than of pauper patients removed unrecovered from asylums to private dwellings, to be placed under the care of relatives, or to be boarded with strangers.

In the disposal of the pauper there is necessarily much less freedom of action than in the disposal of the private insane. In the first place, in the removal of the latter from asylums there are no official authorities whose sanction must be obtained. In the removal of paupers, on the other hand, the concurrence of the parochial authorities and of the superintendent of the asylum is required. In this impediment lies, I believe, one of the chief causes of the proportionally

smaller number of pauper removals. A relieving officer
who has his pauper lunatics safely lodged in the asylum,
is free from any further responsibility connected with
them. Their maintenance is defrayed by the Union,
and as their discharge would only increase his cares,
he not unnaturally discourages all proposals to this
effect.

In the second place, the circumstances of the families
of the pauper insane naturally limit choice. An insane
inmate in a family is not only a source of direct ex-
penditure, but very frequently, from the supervision
which he requires, a source of diminished income.
Hence in many cases a great unwillingness to receive
him. But whether these surmises are right or wrong, it
is very certain that the different degrees in which the
private and pauper insane accumulate in asylums are
due to artificial causes, and are not inherent in the
malady *per se.*

It is upon the preceding views that recent lunacy
legislation in Scotland has been conducted. Increased
facilities have been given for the discharge of pauper
patients from asylums, and for their accommodation
in private dwellings, in numbers which must not, however, exceed four in any one house. On the 1st of
January, 1866, the number of pauper lunatics so placed
was 1568, and their condition is stated by the Commissioners to have been on the whole very satisfactory.
Many of them were industrially employed in farm
operations, household work, as messengers, &c.; and so
carefully had their selection been made, that no accident

of a serious character is known to have occurred to any pauper lunatic living in a private dwelling under the sanction of the Commissioners, since the institution of the Lunacy Board. The rate of mortality in 1865 was only 5·3 per cent., and was even less in former years; a result which of itself affords conclusive evidence of general good treatment.

Young imbecile women, with active erotic tendencies, are placed in asylums; and it appears that practically among the fifteen to sixteen hundred *selected* patients, whose management in private dwellings has received the sanction of the Board, the risk of pregnancy has been exceedingly small—so small as not to be looked on as any objection to the system.

The patients who are thus disposed of are for the most part either congenital idiots, or lunatics affected with dementia or chronic mania, such as are found encumbering the wards of all our large asylums. Many patients of this class require no special treatment; and indeed while in the asylum are left, with scarcely any superior supervision, under the care of attendants, whose rule, in my opinion, is less likely to be humane than that of the occupants of private dwellings, if for no other reason than the greater number which the former have to control, and the more unnatural circumstances in which both they and their patients are placed. The statutory provision made for the supervision of pauper lunatics in private dwellings in Scotland consists in visits made twice a year by the Inspector of Poor, four times a year by the parochial

medical officer, and once a year by the Commissioners
in Lunacy. Annual Reports are made on each case by
the Commissioners to the Board of Lunacy, by whom
the removal of the patient to an asylum is instantly
required, when the report of their condition is unsatisfactory. There can be no doubt that this system of
accommodation in private dwellings is much more
natural than that which is provided by asylums; but
much of its ultimate success will depend on the provision which parishes may be disposed to make for the
maintenance of the patients. Unless it be liberal, there
will be a lack of proper food and clothing, and a limit
in the choice of guardians which will prove disastrous;
for guardians must be sought not among the wretchedly
poor, but among those who have clean and comfortable
dwellings. Much will also depend on the co-operation
of the superintendents of asylums, for, without the sti-
mulus of their recommendation to remove the patients,
many inspectors of poor, for the reasons already stated,
will prefer to leave their patients in confinement. For
further details of the working of the system we refer
to the Annual Reports of the Scotch Commissioners
in Lunacy, and to Dr. Arthur Mitchell's work, *The
Insane in Private Dwellings.*

My opinions, then, regarding the propriety of dis-
posing of a certain class of the insane in private
dwellings, are in great measure founded on the system
of careful selection and supervision, which has been
adopted by the Board of Commissioners in Lunacy for
Scotland. The plan must not be judged of by what

exists in other countries. In France, for instance, where there are upwards of fifty thousand (53,160) lunatics disposed of in this manner, they are left, I believe, without any supervision.

In England there are nearly seven thousand (6638) of the insane poor in private dwellings, regarding whose condition, we are told, the Commissioners have but little information. It is only necessary, however, to read the Annual Reports of the English and Scotch Commissioners to feel satisfied that an official surveillance over those of the insane, who are not in· asylums, is, and probably always will be, much needed. Under an efficient inspection and well-considered regulations, it is clear that the condition of the insane thus disposed of can be ameliorated, and may, perhaps, be made so satisfactory as to justify an extension of the system. Apart from this last consideration, however, the official inspection alluded to would yield an important result in affecting the removal to asylums of patients unsuitable for private dwellings,—those, for instance, who are deemed curable under asylum treatment; or those who have suicidal tendencies, and for whose protection the appliances of an asylum are needed; or those who are dangerous and violent, and who cannot be safely kept at home without restraint; or those whose peculiar habits, erotic propensities, or physical infirmities, make it difficult to manage them properly in private dwellings. The mere withdrawal of such patients would necessarily make the condition of the class as a whole more satisfactory, but it seems certain, from what has been done

H

in Scotland, that the condition of those whose mental
or bodily state does not unfit them for home treatment,
may in various ways be improved.

With reference to the large number of the insane
who are in private dwellings in France, the propriety
and need of official supervision have been well pointed
out by M. Falret. He says :—"Du reste, alors même
que le nombre des aliénés conservés dans leurs familles
ne serait pas augmenté et resterait ce qu'il est au-
jourd'hui, il y aurait encore là un côté de la bien-
faisance publique relative aux aliénés qui mériterait au
plus haut degré de fixer l'attention des médecins et de
l'administration. Il y a évidemment, sous ce rapport,
une lacune dans l'appui et la protection que l'Etat doit
aux aliénés non séquestrés, à leurs familles, et à la
société. Ces aliénés méritent, comme les autres, qu'une
administration paternelle veille sur eux, sur leurs in-
térêts, sur leur sécurité, et sur les soins qui leur sont
donnés par leurs familles. On devrait donc créer une
inspection officielle pour les aliénés laissés en liberté
dans leurs familles, comme il y en a une pour les aliénés
séquestrés."[1]

It is then very generally admitted that there is a certain number of the insane who do not require the
special appliances of an asylum for their proper care
and treatment, and who derive enjoyment from the
greater freedom and more natural conditions of domestic
life. "I cannot but think," says Dr. Maudsley in his
recent work on the Physiology and Pathology of the

[1] *Annales Médico-Psychologiques*, March, 1865, p. 254.

Mind, already referred to,[1] "that future progress in
the improvement of the treatment of the insane lies
in the direction of lessening the sequestration and
increasing the liberty of them. Many chronic insane,
incurable and harmless, will be allowed to spend the
remaining days of their sorrowful pilgrimage in private
families, having the comforts of family life, and the
priceless blessing of the utmost freedom that is com-
patible with their proper care."

Dr. Mitchell, in the work referred to, expresses
similar views. "It is clear," he says, "that continued
confinement may be an injury to many of those patients
for whom the appliances of an asylum have ceased to
be necessary, and that, under proper arrangements,
their removal may become the source of increased comfort, happiness, and well-being;" and as evidence of this
he points to the "greater chance of living which we
know they acquire by removal to more natural or less
artificial surroundings."[2]

Indeed, much of the marvellous change for the
better, which has taken place in our asylums may be
regarded as originating in the opinion that considerable
liberty may be safely accorded to many of the insane.
"For the last 70 years," says M. Falret, "reform in
asylums has consisted in a progressive departure from
hospitals and prisons, and in an approach as close
as possible to ordinary dwellings and to ordinary family
life."[3] It seems little more than an extension of this

[1] Page 430.
[2] *Insane in Private Dwellings*, by Dr. Mitchell, p. 80.
[3] *Annales Médico-Psychologiques*, Jan. 1865, p. 95.

to admit the propriety of providing, for some of the insane, the comforts and amenities of *actual family life.* That it is possible to do so with safety and propriety in many cases, may be seen in what has been accomplished in Scotland. The only class of the insane in England who are in private dwellings and under careful supervision are the Chancery patients, and with reference to them Dr. Maudsley writes: — "I have the best authority for saying that their condition is eminently satisfactory, and such as it is impossible it could be in the best asylum."

Professor Griesinger, when alluding to the question in his *Mental Pathology and Therapeutics,* already quoted, says that it has been proved "that the greater number of the insane do not require the confinement of an asylum; that many of them can safely be trusted with more liberty than these institutions allow; and that association in the family life is very beneficial to many of the insane." Dr. Conolly also seems to have contemplated, at an early period, that a certain class of the insane should be out of asylums. In the last chapter of his *Indications,* he appears to have thought that they would be the "majority"; [1] and he proposes in reference to them a careful system of supervision. He gives it as his opinion that "no patient should be confined in a lunatic asylum, except on the particular representation of the relatives or friends that he could not have proper care and attention out of it." [2] Dr.

[1] P. 483.   [2] P. 481.

Conolly uses the term *restraint* in a wide sense and as applicable to much more than mechanical appliances, and he is at pains to point out that it is only just to certain of the insane that they should not be confined in an asylum,—extending this even to those labouring under some forms of insanity which are deemed curable.[1]

In a letter from Dr. Jarvis, dated March 10th, 1869, he says, " The thought is entertained and gaining ground in America, that many of the insane may be better managed out of than in hospitals, and this opinion is beginning to be acted on."

[1] P. 423-4, p. 428-431, p. 373.

XI.

DR. CONOLLY long perceived the want of a lunatic asylum for the middle classes in the vicinity of London, where he knew from experience that such an asylum was greatly needed. At a public meeting, called for the purpose of promoting this object, he made the following statement to show the want of such an institution :—" My connection with the large asylum at Hanwell constantly brings to my knowledge cases for which no suitable asylum yet exists ; and if time permitted, I could cite heart-rending instances of the distress and grief brought on respectable families from this cause."

And on another similar occasion he remarked :—

" Great and liberal provision is made not only in this county, but throughout the kingdom generally, for the reception and care of the pauper lunatic ; and although no one was more alive than he was from experience to the distressing condition of the rich when insanity overtook them, still institutions existed in which they might be received. But between the richer classes and the pauper there was a large class, whom it was difficult to designate properly, but who were generally, for distinction's sake, called the middle class.   That class comprehended persons of education and respectability, whose means of living depended on their own exertions, and the moment they were struck with insanity their means of livelihood were cut off, and they became in reality more helpless than the poor. Such a condition as this, in which the middle class were placed, was as distressing as any they could well conceive, as no provision was made for such cases."

Dr. Conolly exerted himself to the utmost to accomplish an object which he had much at heart; but although he was ably supported by Lord Shaftesbury and other influential noblemen and gentlemen, in addition to the support and interest of his professional friends, he failed to interest the public in the case. Not disheartened by his failure, he made a second attempt some years afterwards, but with no better result.

Many other physicians have witnessed and described the distress occasioned in families when one of the members became insane. Such cases cannot often be properly treated at home, and the means of the family are totally inadequate to enable them to avail themselves of a private asylum. Thus it frequently happens that the period when treatment is of most consequence is lost, and what might by early judicious treatment have been a temporary attack, may prove permanent, and the unfortunate patient become a source of affliction to, and a burden on, the family for life.

The benefits of early treatment in a well-appointed

asylum are too rarely accorded to this class, and the
worst of the only two possible courses is followed.
Rather than place such patients among actual paupers,
even when this can be done, their friends keep them at
home, where restraint and seclusion must frequently be
resorted to, while the disease is in its acute state. We
know little of what the results of early treatment in
private dwellings might be if well conducted; but we
know too certainly that treatment such as I have
alluded to, under circumstances so unfavourable, must
generally end, wherever it is practised, in confirming
the patient's malady, and too often extinguishing the
hope of cure. It would be an act of the highest philanthropy to create and endow (by public subscription, or
by individual munificence) middle class institutions,
in which such patients could be received at low rates of
board, paid of course by themselves or by their friends,
and not by parochial Boards.

Mr. Gaskell, one of the Commissioners in Lunacy, a
man of the largest experience in everything regarding
the treatment of lunatics, expresses himself in the
strongest terms on the " urgent need of accommodation
for the insane of our middle classes." Dr. H. Munro and
Dr. Maudsley have also expressed their opinion in
strong terms on the necessity of such asylums; and
Dr. Lockhart Robertson, the able Medical Superintendent of the Sussex County Asylum, published a
pamphlet urging the establishment of a middle class
asylum in Sussex. Lord Shaftesbury, than whom no

one is better acquainted with the state of lunacy and lunatic establishments in this county, is equally urgent in pressing the great need of such middle class institutions.

In 1857 his Lordship published a letter, in which he urges the necessity of asylums for the middle classes under the inspection of the Commissioners in Lunacy, and describes, in feeling terms, the great misery entailed on families when one of the members is attacked with insanity.

At a later period Dr. Conolly had the gratification of promoting by his influence the establishment of the *Coton Hill Asylum*, near Stafford. This asylum is conducted on the same principles originally proposed by Dr. Conolly for middle class asylums, and it is in every respect admirably adapted for all the purposes of such an institution. *Barnwood House*, near Gloucester, is another excellent asylum conducted on the same principles. These asylums, although established chiefly for the middle classes, are not limited to them; they also receive patients in affluent circumstances, but no one derives any profit from them. The surplus of the payments of the more wealthy patients, after defraying the cost of their maintenance, goes partly to lighten the payment of the patients whose means are straitened. No paupers are admitted; but at this moment I understand there are not a few in both asylums who pay less than their maintenance costs. When the debt incurred in establishing these institutions is liquidated,

the whole surplus will go to reduce the payments.
These asylums are an unspeakable boon to persons of
education and refinement, often literally without any
means—clergymen, professors, and literary men, gover-
nesses, &c., whose incomes too often cease with the
attack of their disease, and for whom no home is left
but a pauper asylum.

There is an able resident physician in each of these
asylums, and the most approved arrangements are
adopted for the treatment of those cases which admit
of a cure; while for those chronic cases which are
found incurable, everything is done to make the house
as like a private dwelling as is possible. Both these
asylums stand in extensive grounds affording ample
space for exercise and amusement in the open air; and
within doors they are supplied with everything that can
contribute to the occupation and amusement of the
patients—a library, daily newspapers, periodicals, bil-
liard tables, bagatelle boards, &c., &c. Excursions into
the country are made almost daily in fine weather, and
many of the patients spend several weeks in the summer
at the seaside. These two asylums are given as
examples of what asylums of this class ought to be. No
restraint is used in them—kindness and gentleness
characterise the whole treatment. It is greatly to be
desired that the number of institutions conducted on
such principles, and serving such a useful and benevolent
purpose, should be increased.

At Nottingham there is an excellent asylum conducted

upon the same principles as these two; and there is a county fund, which reduces the rates at which the poor inhabitants of the county are received.[1]

There is a class of lunatic asylums in Scotland admitting both pauper and paying classes which are very useful.

Seven large institutions of this class exist, and have long existed in Scotland, and they at present afford accommodation for between 800 and 900 private, and between 1700 and 1800 pauper patients.

They are usually called chartered asylums, because each has a royal charter of incorporation. They are not designed solely for the reception of pauper patients, but for the reception also of those whose means enable them to defray the expense of care and treatment suitable to a higher station in life. They likewise afford some assistance to patients in reduced circumstances, who from their previous habits can appreciate, but are not able to pay for, a better style of accommodation. The rule, however, is that private patients at pauper rates receive the same treatment, and occupy the same wards as the strictly parochial patients.

These institutions have been erected by funds derived from legacies, subscriptions, and donations, and have

---

[1] There are, I understand, eleven such establishments in England, accommodating altogether about 500 patients, conducted on similar principles as those which have been mentioned; but many others are wanted.

afterwards been extended by additional contributions. The buildings, furniture and grounds being provided, they become self-supporting—the payments made for patients covering all current expenses, and leaving a surplus, which is laid out on extensions of the buildings or grounds, when these are required.

The management is conducted by Boards of Directors, appointed under the charters of incorporation, consisting of directors *ex officio*, of life directors, and in some instances of annual directors, elected at the yearly meeting of contributors. The immediate superintendence is entrusted to physicians of high standing in their profession, who reside on the premises, and have one or more medical assistants, according to the size of the establishment.

Those English institutions which may be regarded as most closely analogous to the chartered asylums of Scotland, are the *Hospitals for the Insane*. The Scotch chartered asylums now practically fulfil the functions of the English county asylums, or their equivalents the Scotch district asylums, receiving pauper lunatics at fixed rates from the districts in which they are situated, and also from other districts, unprovided with asylum accommodation, with which they may have entered into contracts. In addition to this, they of course still continue to afford extensive public provision for the care and treatment of those of the insane who are not paupers, and who may belong either to the affluent or to the middle classes of society.

In no class of asylums in Great Britain is the principle of *non-restraint* more fully accepted, or more thoroughly put into practice, and the whole treatment of the patients is in strict conformity with the requirements of humanity and science.

XII.

THE following interesting account of the origin of
asylums in this country for the protection of idiots and
training of imbecile children, more especially of the
establishment of our National Training Asylum at
Earlswood, I owe to the kindness of Dr. Langdon
Down, the able Medical Superintendent of that model
Institution, the greater part in his own words. Dr.
Down justly remarked that a sketch of Dr. Conolly's
life would be incomplete without some account of the
part which he took in the foundation and development
of the *Earlswood Asylum.* For the idea of that asylum
the country is indebted to *Mrs. Plumbe,* of London.
That lady, led by peculiar circumstances to think much
on the need of a training institution for the feeble-
minded, set to work earnestly to establish one. She
applied in the first instance to Dr. Conolly for information and advice on the subject; and urged him, if
he approved of her object, to co-operate with her in the
establishment of a training asylum for such cases. She
could not have applied to a better person, or one more
ready or capable of advising her in every respect. Dr.
Conolly agreed in the necessity existing for such a
charity, referred to what had been done in that direc-

tion in Paris, and expressed his willingness to work heartily with her in carrying out so excellent an object.[1] Mrs. Plumbe also wisely sought the aid of her pastor, the Rev. Dr. Andrew Reed, already noted for his success in promoting the establishment of charitable institutions. She likewise obtained some useful information from Mr. Gaskell, then Medical Superintendent of the Lancaster Lunatic Asylum, afterwards one of the Commissioners in Lunacy. Still Mrs. Plumbe met with many obstacles, but with the characteristic energy of her sex, she persevered till she attained the object on which she had set her heart; and now she must find her full reward in the contemplation of the present flourishing condition of the noble *Asylum at Earlswood*, and the other similar institutions to which it has given and is giving rise in this country.

Dr. Conolly and Dr. Reed set earnestly to work, and the result of their exertions in the cause of the weak minded and helpless idiot, was the establishment of an institution which will perpetuate their names as philanthropists to future ages. They were ably assisted by Charles Gilpin, Esq., M.P., Mr. Alderman Wire, Sir George Carrol, and other philanthropic men who took a warm interest in the formation of the asylum. Death has removed many of these, but their places have been filled by others who have been animated by their ex-

[1] Dr. Conolly had visited Paris in 1845, and made himself thoroughly acquainted with the state of their institutions for lunatics and idiots. Of this visit he published a full and very interesting account in the *British and Foreign Medical Review*, vol. xix.

ample; and for many years past the Board of Management has been ably seconded in its labours by its zealous Secretary, Mr. Nicholas.

Sir John Forbes became a member of the Board of Management in 1849, and was a frequent attendant at its meetings, up to two years before his death, giving his friend Dr. Conolly the advantage of his constant support in establishing this asylum, as he had done through all his anxious labours at Hanwell. On the 27th of October, 1847, this Institution was established. Park House at Highgate, and afterwards Essex Hall, Colchester, were used for a time, but they were merely temporary habitations. Earlswood near Redhill, Surrey, was selected as the permanent site of the asylum. The foundation stone was laid by the lamented Prince Consort, on the 6th of January, 1853, and opened by His Royal Highness on the 5th July, 1855; and on the 22nd of October, 1858, Earlswood became the seat of the National Asylum for feeble-minded children and idiots. The good work, thus inaugurated, has not failed to fructify. At present, in addition to the Earlswood Asylum, there have been established the following *Idiot Asylums* in Great Britain.

The Bath Asylum.—This small asylum was founded in 1846, by Miss White, who has thus the merit of having established the first training school for feeble-minded children in this country.

The Baldovan Asylum, near Dundee, founded in 1853.

The Asylum at Larbert, near Falkirk, founded in 1859.

The Eastern Counties Asylum, Essex Hall, Colchester, established in 1859.

The Western Counties Asylum, Star Cross, Devon, founded in 1863.

A Northern Counties Asylum is in process of formation at Lancaster, on the model of Earlswood.

An attempt is also being made to establish an asylum in Ireland. These may be considered as some of the fruits of the labours of Dr. Reed and Dr. Conolly in providing for the imbecile.

The subjoined note from Dr. Conolly to Mr. Charles Reed, the son of Dr. Reed, came into my hands when the account of Earlswood was ready for the press. It speaks so highly for the characters of these two remarkable men, that the principal part of it is given below. It has reference to the request of the Editor of a Medical Journal to Dr. Conolly to write a notice of Dr. Andrew Reed. The letter is dated Feb. 12th, 1864.

After thanking Mr. Reed for a memoir of his father, he continues :—" Before I fell into this declining state, nothing would have been so gratifying to me as to endeavour to portray the leading features of the late Dr. Reed's remarkable character in one of our medical publications ; but to do so required time which I could scarcely command, and energy which I felt I no longer possessed. The devotion of a life to the relief of various forms of affliction, and the capacity of so influencing his fellow creatures as to establish so many permanent forms for their relief, were subjects not to be slightly

I

treated, and to describe the combination of qualities
which would have distinguished Dr. Reed, as a statesman, with the sensibility of temperament which is
evinced in so many passages in his writings and in his
life; the great practical power, with the calm perseverance maintained in all difficulties,—the practical
philosophy, indeed, and the ever present and deep
religious feeling animating and sustaining all that he
did, and his constant examination of himself; these
and other traits of his great character—not to speak
of his extraordinary exertions and influence as a divine,
—would be a task which, after all, could never be accomplished so well as it has been done in the 'Memoir'
by his sons.

"I shall always reflect with pleasure in having been
permitted to share, although in a very small degree, in
Dr. Reed's labours in the cause of the Idiot; his bright
example is at this time suggesting like efforts in Ireland
and in other countries. If his valuable life had been
prolonged, I believe he would have assisted me in
endeavouring to found a charitable retreat for the insane
of the middle and educated classes, for whom we have
no adequate provision in England. But this is a work
to be done by others, after a few more years—perhaps by
some whom Dr. Reed's bright example may stimulate!"

"With Dr. Reed's, Dr. Conolly's name," writes Dr.
Down, "must for ever remain associated with the history
of Earlswood Asylum, giving to the enterprise at its commencement, not unattended by difficulties, the advantage
of his great name, working diligently for its advance-

ment at the meetings of the Board while his strength
lasted, and up to the latest period of his life animating,
by his sympathy and wise counsel, the active adminis-
trators in their work. It may be safely said that Earlswood would not have attained its present position, but
for the noble qualities of heart and mind possessed by
Dr. Conolly."

The Earlswood Asylum aims to be national in its
scope, and a model for others. Following the efforts
which were made in France and in America, it has produced results, and presents an organisation unequalled
as a training asylum in this or any other country ; and
by its example and success has done much to encourage
the benevolent both at home and abroad, who are seek-
ing to follow in the same path.

By the Annual Report 1867, there were under training at Earlswood 450 inmates; about two-thirds males
and one-third females. They are classified in various
ways in order to establish the possibility of companionship and to facilitate educational effort. Of these about
350 receive daily instruction in the schools, where not
only the usual subjects of education are taught, but
classes are formed for teaching various household duties.
There are in addition extensive workshops, where 150
of the male inmates take parts in various industrial
pursuits, and with such result that a medal has been
awarded by the Jurors, in Class 91 of the Paris Exhibi-
tion, for the specimens of handicraft forwarded by the
institution. Besides these, there is a farm of 150 acres,
with kitchen and pleasure gardens, which furnish pro-

ducts to the house, as well as a means of out-door occupation for those who are physically competent. A
nursery exists for children of tender years, as well as
an infirmary for the sick and feeble. Amusements of
various kinds take place at weekly intervals, which not
only interest the inmates, but prove beneficial to the
staff, on whose mental freshness and vigour the progress and happiness of the patients in a great measure
depend.

All the departments are under medical supervision,
and all are made to subserve *the one object of developing
mental power through improved physical condition.*

The following is an extract of a letter, by Dr. Conolly,
dated Hanwell, Oct. 17th, 1860, addressed to his friend
Dr. Browne, Commissioner in Lunacy for Scotland, urging
the establishment in Scotland of an institution " for the
care and training of the imbecile and idiotic," " these
poor outcasts of society." He then describes the " gratification, not unmixed with wonder," which he felt on a
visit to the " model asylum," as he rightly styles it, at
Earlswood. " The spectacle of 300 children there assembled—each child rescued from solitude and neglect,
from misery, from semi-starvation, from mockery and
persecution—is one that does honour to humanity. The
cleanliness, the order, the comfort of all the apartments ; the extensive grounds and pleasant gardens in
which so many groups of children are generally seen,
some at play, some at work, and all pleased to see the
visitors, whom they approach with confidence and trust,
and even with affection ; the schools in which they are

variously educated, and with never-ceasing patience and kindness; the workshops in which they are taught many useful occupations; the abundant and good food provided for them; the various amusements and re-creations; the large hall in which they meet on dif-ferent occasions, and in which their voices are so often to be heard united in simple prayers, or thanks and devotional song;—all these things combine to give a distinct character to the establishment, as one where goodness and mercy prevail, and to form a scene most impressive upon all who take an interest in the poor creatures, who are the least finished among the works of the great Creator of all things.

" When I remember from what small beginnings all this has arisen, and in how small a number of years, I feel that the practicability of all this good being effected by the appeal of a few earnest and benevolent men to wealthy communities, is so undeniably proved, as to give the fullest encouragement to attempts of a like kind elsewhere."

The following note from Dr. Conolly in reply to one from Mr. Nicholas, Secretary of the Asylum, shews the warm interest he continued to take in the Asylum long after he had been able to visit it. It is dated November 14, 1865 :—

" I am much obliged by your kind letter. It always gladdens me to hear of the prosperity of Earlswood, and of your continued health and usefulness. Twelve months have passed away since I last visited London, and I have no hope of ever again seeing Earlswood.

I hope your own labours will be long and happily continued, and aided by such good men as you have as
yet happily on the Board.   You may believe that it
always gladdens my heart to hear good accounts of the
Rev. Mr. Sidney, and as long as I live I shall feel
interested in whatever is done at Earlswood."

As an appropriate conclusion to this interesting
description of the admirable Asylum at Earlswood, I
subjoin an extract from a letter which I received from
Dr. Down, long before I was aware that I could obtain
from that gentleman so full an account of the establishment as that just given.   It was in reply to my enquiry
regarding the influence of Dr. Conolly's visits, &c., in
the Asylum.

" My knowledge of Dr. Conolly," writes Dr. Down,
" dates only from 1858, and my first interview with him
was when he, Sir John Forbes, and Dr. Little, selected
me from the other candidates for appointment as
Medical Superintendent to Earlswood Asylum.   From
that time no one can be in a better position than myself to judge of Dr. Conolly's work and value in relation
to the institution.

" His visits were the most refreshing incidents of my
recollection in connection with the Asylum.   Entering
on my work as an untried man, and finding myself
allied to an institution which had become unpopular
at the Lunacy Board, I was mainly decided on holding
a position which had so much to overwhelm one, by
the influence of Dr. Conolly.   That influence was
magical.   The humility of his character was only

equalled by the real love he manifested for the mentally afflicted.

"At the visits of the Board of Management, he would
steal away from his colleagues and was to be found
holding loving intercourse with the little members of
my charge, in a way that one has never seen before or
since. Moreover, he so encouraged every official in his
or her work, that the savour of his visit lasted till he
again returned; and who shall estimate the value of
Dr. Conolly's name to the Asylum? I am quite sure
that it would have had difficulty in surmounting its
early trials but for the confidence his name inspired.

"For myself, I have often had to seek his counsel,
and never without being struck with his judgment and
the fascination of his influence, the high resolve he
inspired in one, and what willingness he exhibited to
maintain, co-equally with the responsibility, the power
of the Medical Superintendent, and thus to prevent a
repetition of those evils which he had so bitterly to
lament in his own experience.

"Only a few weeks before his decease I found him,
as ever, ready to aid by his advice, loyal to the honour
of his profession, and singularly unselfish in all his
thoughts and deeds."

It has been very gratifying to the author of this
memoir to find how all who were intimate with Dr.
Conolly agree with Dr. Down's account of his high-
minded, generous, and unselfish character.[1]

[1] When these sheets were preparing for the press, the account of
Dr. Down's resignation reached me. His retirement is a great public

Not the least effective of Dr. Conolly's efforts in the
cause of the insane and the idiot were his eloquent and
influential addresses at public meetings convened for
their support. The following portion of one of those
addresses is given as a specimen; but to fully estimate
his oratorical powers, the influence of that earnest, persuasive language, in which he pleaded the cause of the
unfortunate, it was necessary to hear him speak. As
Sir Thomas Watson has well remarked—"his oratory
was easy, copious, elegant, and persuasive."

At a public meeting held at Cambridge in support
of the Earlswood Asylum, then occupying Essex Hall,
Colchester, the Rev. Mr. Sidney, who has been justly
called the friend of the idiot, addressed the meeting,
giving an interesting account of the principles and
methods pursued in the management and teaching of
the children, and the successful results, ending by
proposing a resolution in favour of supporting the
institution. Dr. Conolly, in seconding the resolution,
said :—

"In these statements are to be found our apology
for appealing to you for assistance in our attempts to

loss. He filled his position in the Earlswood Asylum in a way in
which no man has filled a similar position in this country or in any
country in Europe. I give this not only as my own opinion, but I
believe it to be the general opinion among those who have given
attention to the training of imbecile children. Dr. Down was a
scientific man, and he greatly advanced our knowledge of Idiocy,
and what he did gave promise of much more. He was an earnest,
able, working man, such as it was most desirable to see at the head
of our greatest institution, and in the direction of public opinion on
this subject.

improve the condition of the idiot. We appeal to you, who possess health of body and of mind, to consider the unhappy state of those whose infirmities preclude the perfect possession of either. We come to address you, in a place where the loftiest aspirations of the human intellect have been so many times manifested, to petition for those whose intellectual condition is so low that they are withdrawn from ordinary observation, and are among the most obscure and helpless of mankind. We come to entreat you to look with an eye of pity on many who can never comprehend the extent of your goodness to them, and whose speech and language will never enable them to express their gratitude to you. There must be many in this company to whom the joy of watching the dawn of infant intelligence has been well known, and who have felt the delight of observing the gained attention, the smile of recognition, the little outstretched hand and offered lip of a dearly-loved child; its varied expression of countenance, its pleasure in novel objects, its manner of learning how to use its arms and hands, its growing desire to walk, its marvellous acquisition of the power of attaching sounds and names to things and persons; and all the curious and gradual evolution of the spirit that is within it. Those who have known this pleasure can best imagine a parent's anxious mind, when the contemplation of this progressive development is first interrupted by some *doubt*, arising from the mother's closer and fonder observation, she scarcely knows how, but which fills her with a vague dread respecting her child's actual advancement.

Sometimes she fears that in the little eyes she watches there is not even the speculation of infancy. Again and again the doubt is put aside, and fear and hope again and again succeed each other, until at length she makes the dreadful discovery that her child is an idiot. It is, indeed, a discovery full of cureless woe. For, for that child, what is life to be? A fatuous infancy; a childhood no less helpless than infancy: no power of perfect speech; no natural exercise of its limbs; scarcely a capacity for knowing one person from another. Years proceed, and every year makes the deficiencies of the poor imperfect creature more conspicuous, or perhaps more revolting. It utters loud but scarcely intelligible sounds, and has little or no articulate speech. It laughs —but its laughter communicates no joy. It walks and runs—but a mere animal impulse seems to govern its movements. It learns nothing—not even how to protect itself from danger. Whilst a child, its passions cause distress to those about it: in more advanced years they become more and more the causes of terror. For this poor being, however highly born, all the avenues to use-fulness, and to distinction and fame, are closed. Nay, worse than this, its tendency is to become mischievous, degraded, and disgusting; whilst its limited intelligence shuts it out from all affectionate communion with its brothers and sisters, and all its relatives, and seems to sever them from one another as if for ever, or as a being not of the same species. If the occurrence of an idiotic or imbecile infant is so great a disaster in ranks of life placed above mere toil and the fear of want, what is the result of such a calamity in a poor family, among the classes dependent upon daily industry for daily bread? It is destitution for life. I would ask you to accompany, in imagination, the officers of this charity, or members of its Board, in their visits to these poor creatures at home, and in a London home. An application has been made for the admission of a child to the Asylum; and the object of the application is to be visited, and its state and that of its parents inquired into. After some search, the family is found in some obscure and unhealthy locality, where, from want and ignorance combined, every neglect exists that invites every physical and moral evil; everything that seems to solicit epidemic diseases to settle and spread there, and to ask the cholera to come, and all the scrofulous forms of deterioration to abide, and all the disfigurements of the human form and human mind to manifest themselves. In damp rooms, in close and noisome courts, or in desolate, unventilated apartments, reached by no inviting stair, are to be found residing, and for ever toiling, the parents who have applied for assistance. Parents who have shown this anxiety are usually industrious, but very poor. The father works at some handicraft business, and his wife is engaged in washing, or in some less liberally remunerated work, as shoe-binding, or waistcoat-making, or perhaps shirt-making. They must work or starve. They know no holidays; for if they cease to work, they and their little children must cease to eat; cease to have a fire to warm them, clothes to cover them, or any kind of bed to sleep upon. For

the house seems generally full of little children, not yet
old enough to work, and who are yet unconscious that
their lot in life is mere labour; and whose appearance
is often so delicate and attractive as to form a strange
contrast with the things around them. Nothing has yet
effaced the Divine image from their brows, and their
lips, and their hearts. One little creature there is,
however, in that poor dwelling, which cannot run about
with the rest. That little creature is the object of the
visit. You will find it in winter placed by the fire, and
in summer by the door, seated in a little chair, or lying
in a little bed. It gazes upon its livelier brothers and
sisters with the peculiar expression of imbecility. Its
smile is vacant. It cannot use its limbs, nor get out of
its chair without help, nor keep out of the fire without
watching. It cannot dress itself, nor feed itself, nor
help itself in any way. Without the constant care of
others it must die. But that care presses heavily always,
and ruinously at last, on its poor parents. The matter
of admiration is, that this imperfect little creature,
which only entails privations upon them, is still to them
an object of even peculiarly tender solicitude. The
happier little children of the same family learn the same
feeling; and seem to love their afflicted brother or
sister more than they love one another. They watch it,
they protect it from danger, they try to amuse it, they
draw it about, and they give it some of their own little
portions of food. With increased stature and strength,
however, the necessity of labour comes upon them. One
by one they go from home, and support themselves.

The poor imbecile alone remains, and becomes even a heavier burthen to its father and mother when years are gathering over them. With all that they can do, the child grows only a stronger animal; learns to walk about, but is uninstructed, uncontrolled, helpless; if possessed of much energy, the dread of the neighbours; and if quiet and timid, hunted from street to street, and exposed to every kind of wanton cruelty. Between the two extremes of society which I have mentioned, there are many ranks of life in which parents engaged in various kinds of business, who have the misfortune to have an idiotic or imbecile son or daughter, very painfully feel the difficulty of procuring for them the systematic and special education that they require; and, seeing them grow up untaught, wayward, and incapable of useful occupation, are harassed with bitter thoughts as to the means of providing for them when left behind. Now it is to meet all these forms of destitution that the Asylum for Idiots has been established. All the applicants, of whatever class, are visited, examined, and, as far as the means of doing so yet permit, are finally gathered under the wings of this great Christian charity."

The man who could think and feel in this fashion, and could clothe his thoughts and words in such language, possessed a rare combination of gifts, and it is no marvel that such a man proved a great power among his fellow-men, convincing their judgment, and touching their hearts.

XIII.

FOREIGN ASYLUMS.—The following brief notices of foreign asylums, is introduced here to show the state of these institutions in different countries, as regards the care and treatment of the insane, and more especially with respect to the practice of the non-restraint system.[1]

France.—That non-restraint should not have been at once accepted in the country of Pinel and Esquirol, greatly disappointed Dr. Conolly, and the more so, as he had many esteemed friends among the alienist physicians in Paris, of whose humane feelings towards the insane, and of their earnest desire to improve their treatment, he was well aware. " The principles which guide and animate the good *alienist* physicians of Paris," he remarked, " are evidently identical with those zealously cherished by the non-restraint physicians of England ; and these principles will assuredly lead to perfect conformity of practice. We owe an ancient and great debt to the French in relation to the insane ; and it is to be hoped that they will not think it an unworthy condescension to borrow something from us in return." [2]

---

[1] *For further information on the state of European asylums see Appendix A.*

[2] *Treatment of the Insane without Mechanical Restraints*, p. 366.

The asylum establishments in Paris have lately undergone great and very beneficial improvements.

The old asylums, the Bicêtre and the Salpêtrière, have been lately set apart for the reception of the aged chronic cases of the insane, and for idiots and epileptics. Three new asylums have been erected for the Department of the Seine, each to contain 600 patients,—300 of each sex. Two of the asylums are surrounded with ample grounds for the erection of workshops, for gardening, agriculture, recreation, &c. In each of these establishments there is a department for private patients from the middle classes of society, who pay for their maintenance and treatment. There is a central Bureau in Paris, at which all patients are received, and where they remain for a short time, in order that the character of their disease may be ascertained and they are in a state to be transferred to the asylum destined for them.

The treatment in these hospitals is most humane, restraint is seldom employed, and when it is, the camisole is the only form in use, and even that is seldom resorted to.

The departmental asylums in France, which may be compared to our county asylums, are not, according to reports, in a satisfactory state generally. M. Morel, however, gives us reason to believe that the treatment of the insane in these asylums has improved greatly within the last few years. " Je ne puis toutefois que féliciter mes collègues d'être mieux disposés qu'on ne l'était généralement en France il y a quelques années à peine, pour l'usage de plus en plus limité des moyens restrictifs; c'est là ce que constatent les lettres qui m'ont été adressées de toutes parts." [1]

M. Morel's information is very satisfactory, and there is good reason to believe that the improvement continues to increase.

M. Morel, just cited, an eminent physician of large experience on the subject of lunacy and lunatic asylums, visited England in 1858, with the express object of examining the state of our lunatic asylums, and observing the practice and effects of the non-restraint system of treatment. After a full inspection of our whole asylum system, and a careful examination of the practice of non-restraint in all its phases, he returned to France a convert to the system, and published the excellent work, just referred to, on its advantages, replying, at the same time, to the misconceptions entertained to it by foreign physicians.

To the faithful and clear account which M. Morel has given of the practice and effects of non-restraint, Dr. Conolly expresses his entire satisfaction in the following extract of a letter to his friend, M. Battel, Dec. 23rd, 1860:—

"You will scarcely require to be assured that your letters on the subject of M. Morel's Report were all extremely interesting to me. He has given a most fair and exact account of the system of non-restraint; and has stated everything with such moderation, and with

---

[1] *Le Non-Restraint, ou De l'Abolition des Moyens exercitifs dans le Traitement de la Folie,* Paris, 1860, par M. le Docteur Morel, Médecin-en chef de l'Asile de *Saint-Yon* (Seine-Inférieure).

such candid acknowledgment of various difficulties
as will, I trust, conciliate even those who yet oppose
his views.   I am myself satisfied with a firm belief that
eventually the physicians of France will condescend to
follow us islanders in this part of treatment.   You have
yourself been the first to attract attention to this subject
in France, and I admire your candour in representing it,
and your judgment in not attempting to force it on the
attention of the eminent physicians of Paris."

With the view of shewing M. Morel's opinion of non-
restraint, and the calming effect it produces in our
asylums, I have taken the liberty of making several
extracts from his work, which the interest M. Morel
takes in the subject will lead him, I hope, to excuse.

After citing two remarkable cases illustrative of the
effects of the non-restraint system in calming two furious maniacs treated by Dr. Hitchman, in the Derbyshire Asylum, and who ultimately recovered, M. Morel
gives the following instructive case which occurred in
the Bicêtre :—

"À l'appui de ces deux faits, j'en citerai un troisième
qui les corrobore, et qui m'a été révélé par *M. Battel*,
ancien administrateur des hospices de Paris.   En 1847,
ce fonctionnaire visitait l'asile de Bicêtre avec le *fils du
docteur Conolly*.   Un aliéné violent, attaché depuis plu-
sieurs jours sur le fauteuil de force, vociférait d'une
manière incessante, et la salle où il était retenu retentis-
sait de ses formidables cris.   Le surveillant de service
déclarait qu'on ne pouvait sans danger lui laisser la
liberté de ses mouvements.   L'administrateur demanda

K

alors à M. Conolly ce que ferait son père si un tel
malade était confié à ses soins. 'Il ferait,' répondit ce
jeune homme, 'ce que je vais faire moi-même si vous
voulez me le permettre. Il couperait immédiatement
les liens de cet infortuné, et le laisserait à ses impul-
sions en le faisant convenablement surveiller.' Cette
tentative valait la peine d'être faite; le malade fut
aussitôt détaché. A peine affranchi de ses entraves, il se
promena dans le préau de la manière la plus paisible et
la plus inoffensive, adressant de vifs remercîments à ceux
qui l'avaient affranchi de la torture à laquelle il était
soumis. *Quinze jours après, il sortait guéri de l'asile.*[1]

"Dans son dernier rapport de 1849, dix années après
la promulgation du *non-restraint*, M. le docteur Conolly,
énumérant tous les avantages moraux qui sont résultés
pour cet asile de l'introduction du *non-restraint*, ajoute
ces mémorables et consolantes paroles, que je suis
heureux de transcrire comme un encouragement pour
tous ceux qui voudront entrer dans la même voie : 'Je
veux simplement établir, que dans cet grand asile, point
n'a été besoin depuis dix ans d'attacher un seul pied,
une seule main, soit pendant le jour, soit pendant la
nuit, pour se rendre maître des malades violents ou
désespérés. (No hand or foot has been fastened for the
control of the violent or the despairing.) Aucun instrument de coërcition mécanique (mechanical-restraint)
n'a été employé ou introduit dans les divisions des
aliénés pour quelque cause que ce soit. Aucun patient

[1] *Op. citat.*, p. 45.

n'a été placé dans la chaise de force pendant le jour, ou
fixé dans son lit. Les aliénés les plus excités et les plus
incoërcibles en apparence, à leur entrée à l'asile, ont
été immédiatement débarrassés de leurs liens, et jamais,
depuis, on n'a eu recours envers eux à des moyens coër-
citifs. Je désire ne rien exagérer, mais je dois constater
que le résultat du système a été, pour chaque nouvelle
année commençante, une augmentation dans la tran-
quillité générale et une diminution dans les dangers
que peut faire courir la réunion de plus de mille aliénés.
L'influence salutaire exercée par la nouvelle méthode
sur les malades entrants, même sur les plus violents,
a été telle que le spectacle des terribles formes de
la manie et de la melancolie a formé une bien rare
exception, et que l'ordre de l'établissement n'en a
pas été troublé, ni l'aspect riant qu'il offre nullement
contristé."

" Une chose préoccupe encore les médecins aliénistes
françaiset—cela ressort de toutes les lettres que j'ai
·reçues—c'est la substitution d'un moyen de contrainte à
un autre. Ils ne veulent à aucun prix remplacer la
camisole par la séclusion ou par les bras des infirmiers, et en cela ils ont raison. Mais ce que j'ai dit de
la condamnation de ces moyens par M. Conolly suffit
pour justifier les médecins anglais. Je ne voudrais pas
me répéter ; je ne puis que renvoyer aux détails dans
lesquels je suis entré à propos de l'abus que l'on peut
faire des moyens destinés à remplacer ou à mitiger le
non-restraint."

Dr. Conolly replied long since to these objections to
non-restraint. . Seclusion was never used by him as a
substitute for restraint, but on its own account and then
for very short periods. On the contrary he pointed out
in the strongest terms, in his Reports, and in several
portions of his work, the evils caused by the abuse of
seclusion. He employed seclusion in the mildest
manner and seldom for a longer period than a few
hours, and he recommended it to be preceded, when
possible, by active walking exercise in the open air;
after which he found the soothing effects of seclusion
were more speedily attained.

No doubt in the early stage of the introduction of
non-restraint, seclusion was improperly used in some
asylums contrary to the strict injunctions of Dr. Conolly,
but that practice no longer exists, and in many asylums
active walking exercise in the grounds of the asylum
is made a substitute for it, as has long been the case in
the Montrose Asylum.

"Que font maintenant, je le demande, au milieu
du concert unanime qui règne en Angleterre, les oppositions que l'on peut citer? Ces oppositions, il faut
bien l'avouer, sont la plupart du temps parties d'institutions particulières qui, ne disposant pas d'aussi grandes
ressources que les établissements publics, ne peuvent
arriver aux mêmes résultats. Mais elles n'ébranlent en
rien le principe sur lequel est basé le *non-restraint;*
car, ainsi que je n'ai cessé de le dire, ce principe n'est
pas une chose isolée, une exagération, une affaire de
sentimentalisme ; c'est l'expression de toutes les améli-

orations qui constituent la vie d'un asile, et M. Conolly a eu raison de dire que *restriction et négligence étaient synonymes.*" [1]

Germany. — Dr. Ludwig Meyer, Physician to the lunatic asylum at Göttingen, has the honour of being the first to adopt the non-restraint system of treatment in Germany. After having visited the English asylums, he adopted it, under great difficulties, in the asylum at Hamburgh of which he was Medical Superintendent.[2] Dr. Meyer was soon followed by Dr. Staltz, of Hall, Tirol, who introduced non-restraint into the asylum under his care, and without, it appears, being aware of Dr. Meyer's having previously done so. We are also able to adduce Professor Griesinger of Berlin, as an ardent supporter of non-restraint. Dr. Griesinger, after careful observation of the system as practised in England, convinced himself of its great advantages, and as the following extracts from his excellent work on Insanity will shew, he is now a zealous advocate for its general adoption.

"In taking," Professor Griesinger writes, "a retrospect of the arguments for and against it, we can easily understand how the value of the system of non-restraint was so long questioned, and how the arguments against it appeared to keep the ascendancy. But if we consider that these objections proceeded entirely from those who had not practically tested the system of non-restraint

[1] *Op. citat.*, p. 55.
[2] Dr. Meyer wrote an able article in favour of the system in the *Allgemeine Zeitschrift für Psychiatrie, Siebentes Heft,* 1862.

and had never even witnessed it, their force will not appear so great. If we interrogate experience, which is the only proper test, we shall find that during the last ten years all doubts in reference to it have been removed. The question is now decided entirely in favour of non-restraint. This great reform is now carried out with the most favourable results in every public asylum in England, and the name of *Conolly* will always be mentioned with that of *Pinel,* whose work he has completed.[1]

"Up to the time of the publication of the *first* edition of this work, I allowed myself, influenced by the adverse opinions of the German psychologists, to oppose the system of non-restraint, although at heart I sympathised with the reforms, yet I could not see my way clear to refute the contrary arguments which were advanced. Since then practical experience, from one end of England to the other, has done so. I have seen the new system carried out in several of the large English institutions and have been *convinced.*

"In Hanwell, with a population which has gradually increased till now it reaches about 1000, *for* 21 *years there has not been a hand or foot bound either by night or by day.* Colney Hatch, a very large asylum (1200 patients) was opened in 1849, and never to this day has any means of restraint been employed."

"Compare with this the number who are confined in

[1] *Mental Pathology and Therapeutics,* by W. Griesinger, M.D., &c. Translation by Dr. C. Lockhart Robertson and Dr. James Rutherford. London, 1867, p. 492.

cells—many with strait-jackets,[1] and others actually
reconciled to their sojourn through its long continuance
— in some of our continental asylums where non-
restraint seems to be regarded as a mere chimera. And
let it no more be repeated that such a system is suited
only to the English, who submit more easily to control
than the patients on the continent. Before the time of
Conolly it was believed in England also, that it was
impossible to treat the insane without powerful means of
restraint " (p. 494).

" Let us then pursue with confidence the new system,
fearlessly break off the old practice, and assume new
responsibilities, ever bearing in mind that the least
negligence will re-open the door to the employment of
violence.

" We doubt not that ere long in every new institution
for the treatment of the insane erected in Germany, with
the very foundation-stone the assurance will be laid,—
that for all time to come, the system of non-restraint
only shall be practised within its walls" (p. 495).

Dr. Griesinger's opinion thus strongly expressed
is highly creditable to his candour and philanthropy,
and cannot fail to produce a deep impression on his
medical brethren throughout the whole of Germany.[2]

Italy.—Several English physicians have of late
years (1857-1865) visited the establishments for the

[1] Estimated at 50,000 over the whole of the continent by Baron
Mundy, see p. 191.
[2] For the state of the lunatic asylums in Germany see Appendix A.

insane in Italy. They speak of the physicians of the asylums as generally acquainted with the improvements in the treatment of the insane in this country, and in many instances disposed to abolish entirely all forms of mechanical restraint. But they want the aid of the Government to improve the buildings which are generally ill-suited for the proper treatment of insane patients, and a larger and better staff of attendants, so as to enable them to put the non-restraint system into practice. At present mechanical restraint prevails in most of the asylums of Italy, differing, however, greatly in the extent to which it is employed in different asylums. Dr. Biffi of Milan, for instance, is said to have abolished it entirely in the private establishment which he conducts in the suburbs of that city. At Venice again, Dr. C. L. Robertson and Dr. Howden found the male asylum (placed in the Island of St. Servolo, under the charge of a fraternity of monks), in excellent order: it was clean and apparently well conducted. They saw no indications of restraint, and were told by the physician that it was scarcely ever employed.

On the other hand, the female asylum attached to the General Hospital is described as wretched in the extreme. "Poor women were seen lying in bed, not only handcuffed, but also with anklets secured by a strap to the foot of the bed." [1]

But the two most wretched asylums in that part of Italy, seem to be those of Verona and Brescia, as described by Dr. Arlidge.

[1] *Journal of Mental Science.*

The large asylum in Florence is in a bad state and greatly overcrowded. Mechanical restraint is freely used. Dr. Arlidge observed twenty-five patients under restraint during the day, and the number was no doubt increased during night.[1] Dr. Howden gives the following sad description of the treatment pursued in this asylum : —" Handcuffs, &c., were to be found here as elsewhere ; but the form of restraint which reigned pre-eminent was that of chairs, the construction of which is somewhat peculiar, and certainly very effectual. It is formed like a large arm-chair, from the front of which a board slants down to the ground. In this slanting board are two holes. The patient's legs of necessity rest on this board, and by means of the two holes they are very effectually strapped down. In addition to this the patient wears a pair of handcuffs : from all which it will be readily seen that there is little chance of movement. I shall never forget the spectacle that met my eye on entering one of the female wards. Ranged along the wall were half a dozen of these chairs, and in each chair was seated a poor woman." [2]

And this was the hospital in which Chiarugi, an enlightened and philanthropic physician of Florence, was one of the first in Europe to introduce a mild humane treatment of the insane nearly a century ago, by banishing chains, interdicting blows, and putting an end to permanent seclusion. This he did about the

[1] *Journal of Psychological Medicine.*
[2] *Op. citat.* These chairs are said to be from a model formerly used in St. Luke's Asylum, London.

time that Pinel was doing the same thing in the Bicêtre.[1] It is said that this asylum is about to be transferred to a fine position in the vicinity of Florence. With the change of site it is to be hoped there will be a change of treatment.

Rome.—The best part of this asylum was the portion appropriated to females, where Sisters of Charity attend on the patients, and to their care and attention was no doubt due the cleanly condition of the inmates, many of whom seemed busily engaged sewing and making clothing of all kinds under the kindly superintendence of those Sisters. The wards were, for the most part, large, clean, and airy; and the baths were particularly good.[2]

The portion allotted to the male patients was not by any means in a satisfactory state. There was not the same amount of restraint, however, in this asylum as was to be found in many other Italian asylums; but the medical superintendent seemed to look upon the notion of keeping several hundred patients in one

[1] Chiarugi's book, *Sull' Alienazione Mentale,* was published in Florence in 1793.

[2] Dr. Bacon, who visited the Italian asylums, formed a high opinion of the Sisters of Charity, and of their great usefulness as *nurses* in asylums for the insane. "Their presence and moral influence," he says, "are both respected, even by lunatics, and the effect they exerted may be gathered from the fact that they never meet with violence from their patients; and I have more than once seen a furious and ill-tempered lunatic woman obey instantly the gentle touch and ready smile of a Sister of Charity." They make excellent nurses when placed entirely under the direction of the medical superintendent.

house without ever having recourse to restraint as the most preposterous thing he had ever heard of : in fact, regarded it seemingly as an utter impossibility.

Aversa.—Perhaps more interest attaches to the asylum at Aversa than to any other in Italy, from the experiments made in it long since to improve the treatment of the insane by music and otherwise, and still more from the eminence of its present director, Dr. Miraglia, one of Italy's most enlightened physicians.

Dr. Miraglia has distinguished himself by his study of phrenology, and its application to the treatment of the insane, &c.,[1] and by the zeal with which he has cultivated cerebral pathology, as well as by the interest he has taken in the improvement and treatment of the insane generally in his own country. For these reasons, and for his professional eminence, he has received from King Victor Emmanuel the gold medal and cross of St. Maurice, the highest scientific honour which his country can bestow.

With the exception of a new wing lately built upon an excellent plan under the direction of Dr. Miraglia, the buildings at Aversa are old, and some of them very inconvenient.

It would have given us great pleasure to have been able to cite Dr. Miraglia with the Morels and Griesingers, &c., as an advocate of non-restraint ; but although his treatment is characterized by humanity and gentle-

---

[1] *Trattato di Frenologia applicata alla Medicina, alla Giurisprudenza criminale, alla Educazione, alla Morale, &c.* Napoli, 1854.

ness, he still thinks it necessary to retain restraints, which, however, are seldom used. If Dr. Miraglia would visit the public asylums in this country, making himself acquainted with those of Italy and France on his way to England, there is good reason to believe that he would return to Aversa as strong an advocate of *non-restraint*, as his countryman Dr. Tebaldi.

Dr. Tebaldi visited most of the countries of Europe with the special object of examining their lunatic asylums and modes of practice. On the subject of *non-restraint*, he expresses himself as fully impressed with the great practical superiority of the system, and ably disposes of the specious objections to it of many continental physicians. He concludes his observations on the subject thus:—" Non v' ha dubbio, verrà il giorno che il *no-restraint* non sarà più designato come sistema inglese, ma come quello di tutte le colte e civili nazioni." [1]—" without doubt the day will come when non-restraint shall no longer be styled the English system, but be recognised as that of all civilized nations." [2]

I have to add to Chiarugi another Italian friend of the insane, Baron Pisani of Palermo.

---

[1] *Alienati ed Alienisti: Memorie Medico-critiche dell Dottore Augusto Tebaldi.* Torino, 1864.

[2] Tebaldi is now Professor of Medical Psychology in the University of Padua, and Physician to the Lunatic Asylum, which, much to his regret, forms only a part of the Hospital, and is so miserably arranged that he finds it impossible to introduce the non-restraint system of treatment. The same obstacle exists in the greater number of the Italian lunatic asylums, and there the reform must begin. The profession is quite ready.—*Letter from Prof. Tebaldi*, March 22, 1869.

In 1824, when Baron Pisani was appointed adminis-
trator of the insane of Palermo, he found them, as was
generally the case in Southern countries, mixed with
lepers and loaded with chains, their keepers armed with
clubs, which they applied at discretion. Pisani at once
destroyed the chains, burned the clubs, released those
in solitary confinement, and substituted a mild moral
treatment, which he describes in a letter to Dr. Moore
of London (Dec. 11th, 1835). Pisani's whole treatment, as described in that letter, was most judicious
and successful. After some time he introduced occupation, gardening, building, &c., for the men, and indoor
work of various kinds for the women, with music and
dancing once a week.

In 1845, when M. Morel visited Baron Pisani's asylum
at Palermo, he found it in an excellent condition, and
compared it with one of our best asylums, that of
Derbyshire, " être par ses dispositions intérieures et
extérieures, plutôt une maison de plaisance qu'un
séjour destiné à la plus triste des infortunes."

The asylum continues to be conducted on the same
principles, by the present director Cav. G. Somma
Pareles.

Belgium.—The institutions for the treatment of the
insane in Belgium are chiefly under the care of private
individuals and religious associations. Some of these,
in Bruges and Ghent, are stated to be in good condition
and well managed. Many others contain only a small
number of patients, and this with their private cha-

racter, renders difficult the adoption of recent improvements in the treatment of the insane : lunatic asylums may be too small as well as too large for the best treatment of the patients.

Before the appointment of a commission in each arrondissement to inspect the lunatic asylums, the condition of these institutions throughout Belgium is reported to have been deplorable; and although considerable improvements have been effected under the direction of these commissions, much is still wanted to bring them up to the present improved state of asylums for the care and treatment of the insane.

The first public asylum in Belgium was recently erected in Ghent, after a plan of Dr. Guislain, an eminent alienist physician, whom Belgium has lately had the misfortune to lose. It is to be hoped that this asylum may soon lead to others of a like character in different parts of the country.

In Belgium some of the insane are, and have long been, provided for in a way which professes to carry out the principle of non-restraint to its fullest. More than eight hundred lunatics from various parts of the country are boarded with crofters and tradesmen in the Commune of Gheel. The great majority of these lunatics are paupers, but there are a few who are supported by their friends or from their own funds. The colony is under the care of the State, and a special code of regulations has been framed to meet its peculiarities. Its affairs are directed by a physician who has no other duties, and who has the resident medical practitioners as salaried assistants. The patients are understood to live in family with their guardians, and to join, when possible, in the out-door or in-door occupations of the family. Some years ago a small asylum was erected near the village of Gheel, in which patients are kept under observation for some time after their arrival, and to which patients already in the colony, requiring active medical treatment, are removed.

As regards the merits of the mode of treatment pursued at Gheel, conflicting opinions have been expressed. It cannot be said that mechanical restraint is not practised there, nor that the condition of all the patients is satisfactory. But it appears to be admitted that if the patients in whose cases mechanical restraint is resorted to, and those whose condition is considered faulty were removed, the number remaining would still be large.

There is little doubt that the existence of this colony has of late had a considerable influence on professional opinions as to the treatment of the insane, and that this may be seen in the construction of our asylums and in the greater freedom accorded to the patients. It is certainly a suggestive, as well as a remarkable thing, to find so many hundreds of the insane living at large within a single commune for so long a time, without presenting a longer list of accidents than might be expected from the same number in an asylum.

Denmark.—Dr. Sêlemer, Physician of the Lunatic Asylum of Aarhuus, writes that the system of non-

restraint is not adopted in Denmark to the same extent as in England; but his constant exertion is to
reduce it as much as possible. The same treatment,
he believes, is followed in the other two asylums in
Denmark.

Sweden.—The Swedish Government has long directed
its attention to improve the condition of the insane.
In 1858 a law was passed requiring the insane to
be treated with gentleness, — no means of restraint
injurious to the patient physically or mentally being
allowed; and in 1867 it was further required that a
Report should be made of the number of cases subjected
to seclusion in each asylum. In the *Malmö Asylum*
bodily restraint has been entirely abolished for the last
four years, temporary seclusion being the only restraint
resorted to in refractory cases. "It would be impossible," says Dr. Salomon, " to take up the old practice
of strapping up the patients; even the attendants themselves, knowing from experience that patients get worse
from being tied up in horrid jackets with long sleeves.
Good food and kind words are the best means of keeping
lunatics quiet; and they ought to be attached to their
guardians by the soothing bonds of sympathy. The
humane treatment introduced by Dr. Conolly has produced a remarkable effect in the condition of the insane
in this country contrasted with what it was ten years
ago. Calmness and tranquillity in our asylums have
been substituted for noise and excitement." Dr.
Salomon, the Medical Superintendent of the Malmö

Asylum, to whom I am indebted for the above information, is an enlightened physician and earnest advocate of the non-restraint treatment.

Norway.—A large State asylum has been lately built near Christiania. The treatment is said to be directed with humanity by Dr. Sandberg; still restraints are used—the strait-jacket and restraint-chair; and seclusion is employed to a great extent, in some cases for sixteen hours at a time. In Christiania City Asylum restraint is not only employed as a means of treatment, but also as a punishment; as is seclusion also, with or without the shower-bath. This is avowed by the Medical Superintendent Physician, Dr. Wing.[1]

Holland.—Although in Holland the insane are generally treated with gentleness, the example of Dr. Ewarts has not yet been followed in other asylums. Dr. Ewarts, the physician of the well-arranged asylum at Meerenberg, was the first physician on the continent to introduce non-restraint. During his visit to England in 1854 he was so strongly impressed with the advantages of the non-restraint system that he resolved to adopt it on his return. This he has done with great success. The only means of restraint that he has used is the camisole, and that only for some special purpose, as in surgical cases. Since the introduction of non-restraint seclusion is said to have diminished.

[1] Dr. Lauder Lindsay, *Journal of Psychological Medicine*, 1858, vol. ii.

America.—The following brief account of the present state of the lunatic establishments in the United States was partly obtained from a medical friend who lately made a careful inspection of the asylums of the Eastern States of the Union, with the view of making himself acquainted with their construction, management and whole economy;[1] but it is chiefly derived from an eminent alienist physician of the country, fully informed on everything connected with institutions for the treatment of the insane in America. The Reports of the Proceedings of the Association of Medical Superintendents of American Institutions for the Insane have also afforded me useful information.

The State asylums, and other public asylums or hospitals, as they are indifferently called, of the United

---

[1] Dr. Manning,—who was commissioned by the Government of New South Wales to examine and report on the state of lunatic establishments, and the treatment of the insane, as practised in Europe and America, with the view of enabling the Colony to erect and organize asylums, which should possess all the modern improvements and appliances. An architect had preceded Dr. Manning on the same errand. This is highly creditable to the Colony, and shows the attention which is now being paid to the care and treatment of the insane in civilized countries. Dr. Manning has shown by his elaborate and well digested report, that the Government could not have trusted the Commission to a physician more competent to carry out the inquiry.[a]

---

[a] *Report of Lunatic Asylums.* By Fred. Norton Manning, M.D., Sydney, 1868.—BY AUTHORITY.

States, appear to be in a more satisfactory state than similar institutions are in any country of Europe, Great Britain alone excepted. They are generally built on the double corridor system, the block plan being rarely adopted. As a rule they are kept clean and well ventilated, and well supplied with water. The ventilation is generally effected by machinery, a steam-engine being employed to turn a large fan, which forces fresh, pure air, over pipes containing steam at low pressure, and thence through an elaborate series of channels into the wards and small rooms. Warming is also effected by means of air passed over steam or hot water pipes in the basement;—open fire-places being seldom or never adopted.

The American asylums differ from the county and district asylums of England and Scotland in not being erected specially for the benefit of the insane poor, both paying and pauper patients being received into them, and appropriately accommodated and provided for.

The occupations and amusements, in doors and out of doors, differ little from those used in England. Dancing, however, appears less frequent, gymnastics being employed instead. The American lecture-system has found its way also into the asylums—the medical officers, and lecturers from without, giving lectures and readings on various branches of natural philosophy, and other subjects, and several asylums even possess sets of philosophical instruments to illustrate these lectures. The magic-lantern is in very frequent use.

Libraries exist in almost all asylums, which are generally surrounded with ample grounds for exercise and
occupation.

The proportion of attendants to patients varies from
1 to 10, to 1 to 20. Their character seems to differ
much in the different institutions, the women, as a rule,
appearing to be superior to the men.

Each asylum is entirely under the direction of the
medical superintendent, who has the sole control of
the establishment, and of every person employed in it.
He resides in, or close to, the asylum, and his whole
time is given to his duties, and he has medical assistants in proportion to the number of patients under his
care. Whenever this arrangement is departed from,
and a divided authority is substituted, the general
condition of the asylum suffers in every respect, and
not the least evil consequence appears to be an increase
of restraint. The number of patients in an asylum varies
from 200 to 500 ; up to 350, the medical superintendent
has one assistant; over this number, two assistants. No
class of professional men in the United States are held
in higher estimation than the medical superintendents
of asylums, and in the care and treatment of their
patients there can be no better proof of their possessing
the confidence of the public than the fact that there
are, I understand, not more than five private asylums
in the whole Union. All asylums appear to be inspected : for the State asylums, inspectors are appointed
by the State authorities ; for the corporate asylums, by
the respective boards of trustees.

Fortunately for the insane in America, and the character of their asylums, there were no old half-ruined
monasteries and other similar buildings found in the
country, to be converted into asylums for their insane
poor, as has been done in many countries, though such
buildings are quite unfitted either for the purposes of
care or treatment.   These buildings up to this day are
too often found to be the abodes of the unfortunate
insane in many countries of Europe.   The Americans
had to build their own asylums, and this to their credit
they have done well, every new asylum appearing to be
an improvement on those which had been previously
built.   As in other countries, so in America, the
asylums were for many years considered merely as
places of safe-keeping for lunatics.   The first asylum
devoted to the treatment of the insane appears to have
been built at Worcester, in the State of Massachusetts,
in 1836, and placed under the care of the late philanthropic Dr. S. B. Woodward, considered the father of
the humane treatment of the insane in the United
States.

Although there is much to be admired in the condition of their asylums and in the mode of treatment
of the insane adopted in the United States, non-
restraint has not been the guiding principle of their
system.   Seeing the description of the excellent condition of their asylums, it is to be regretted that they
did not advance a step farther and obtain all the
advantages of non-restraint in addition to what the

best conducted system with restraint as a feature can afford. That this has not been done can only be explained by some such reasons as have prevented the adoption of non-restraint in other countries,—its never having been put to the test of experience, and its being condemned without a trial,[1]—at least I have never heard that it had got a fair trial in America.

Restraints are more or less used in every asylum. The camisole, muff, bed and chair straps, and the crib-bed, are the means of restraint most generally employed. These measures, however, appear to be little resorted to in the best asylums, the treatment as a whole being mild and humane.[2]

Seclusion is employed in all asylums, generally for short periods; the number of the secluded does not seem large, still there is reason to believe that it is more extensively used than in England. Padded rooms are not used in America. To some asylums small cottages are attached, and are occasionally used for seclusion, not without the risk of the seclusion, in such cases, being prolonged beyond the proper object of its application as a remedial measure merely.

"In all the arguments for restraint used by American physicians the evils of seclusion are pointed out; but there is, as a rule, more seclusion, notwithstanding

---

[1] See Professor Griesinger on this point, *Memoir*, p. 135.

[2] It is in the poor-houses of Pennsylvania and in other States, where there is no system of inspection, that restraint, in some of its worst forms, is practised.—Manning, p. 120.

the restraint, in American than in English asylums." [1]
There has, indeed, been for some time a desire among
English superintendents to avoid seclusion as much
as possible, and to substitute active walking exercise
instead. According to Dr. Manning,—"The amount
of seclusion in Continental asylums is, as a rule, not
large; but wherever the amount of restraint was found
to be larger than ordinary, the amount of seclusion was
large also." [2] Such arguments as the following, therefore, can no longer be advanced by the opponents of
non-restraint. *" It is no advance to give up restraining
apparatus and substitute frequent and long-continued
seclusion. An individual may really be more comfortable and much better off in the open air with some
mild kind of restraining apparatus on his person, than
he would be in his chamber without it."*

To this it may be answered: as regards seclusion,
that there appears to be more seclusion in American
than in English asylums; and as regards exercise, it
must be conceded that free exercise in the open air,
without the impediment and degradation of any mechanical restraint, is preferable to restraint in the
mildest form.

The following extract from a report of Dr Kirkbride, one of the most enlightened aliénist physicians
of America, may be adduced as expressing the reason
generally entertained by the medical superintendents of
asylums, for not adopting non-restraint in its full import.

---

[1] Manning, *op. citat.*, p. 121.   [2] *Op. citat.*, p. 121.

Dr. Kirkbride is the Medical Superintendent of the Pennsylvania State Asylum at Philadelphia, and a physician of large experience, and high character. In his Report of 1852 he expresses himself thus:—

" No point connected with the treatment of the insane is now more conclusively established than that every such institution (asylum) may be conducted without any mechanical restraint whatever : whether it is expedient to do so under all circumstances, is not so well settled.   To dispense with restraining apparatus entirely, requires that a hospital should be so constructed as to give all the benefits of the most perfect classification—that it should always have full force of tried attendants and abundant means of exercise and occupation in the open air.   This hospital has never owned a strait-jacket, a muff, or a tranquillizing-chair, or any of the still harsher means formerly used, or the novel ones more recently recommended.   With an average population of more than 200, it is rare to have any restraining apparatus in use.   For the whole period of its existence, the average number using it has not exceeded one per cent., and it has frequently happened that for several months together there has been no mechanical restraint used.   When apparatus is used it is either in the form of leather wristbands secured by a belt around the body, soft leather mittens fastened in the same way, a strong dress with the sleeves connected, or the apparatus for confining the patient in his bed.   Although fully impressed with the conviction that the frequent use of the restraining apparatus is a great evil in any hospital for the insane, it has not been deemed necessary to resolve that it should never be used in this institution."

No treatment can be more humane than that of Dr. Kirkbride, and he had but one step to take to obtain all the advantages of non-restraint, and to get rid of the disadvantages of restraint, of which he seems very sensible. With the excellent state of his hospital, he might easily have abolished restraint entirely, even without the aid of the alterations which he proposes in his establishment. No doubt the arrangement he describes would facilitate the adoption of non-restraint, and Dr. Conolly urged its being done where possible; but he had few such aids in his own case, and if the English superintendents had waited till their asylums were fully organized, non-restraint would not have made the progress in England it has done. In all new asylums, it would certainly be very desirable that the internal construction and arrangements should be such as to facilitate classification, and to aid in every possible way in the humane and curative treatment of the patients, whether conducted with or without restraint.

Dr. Kirkbride mentions an objection to restraint which is often overlooked, but is really a very serious one—its injurious moral influence upon the patients generally—and he remarks on "the advantage of doing away, to the utmost possible extent, with even the *appearance* of restraint in an asylum." "This," he adds,

" is the true field for the ingenious, and their efforts
in this way can scarcely do harm." True ! but there
is one way only of getting rid of this very serious
objection to the use of restraints,—to remove them
entirely from the asylum.   It is evident that every
hospital for the insane must have its value as a curative institution diminished, where mechanical restraints
are seen in use in the wards, exciting, irritating, and
alarming those patients, who are not even themselves
restrained ; thus multiplying the evil consequences of
restraint by adding to the distress and humiliation of
the individual coerced the unhappiness of the whole
asylum.[1]   Dr. Meyer of Göttingen says :—" The knowledge that restraining apparatus exists, has a baneful
influence on the more sane of the patients: it gives
them a feeling of insecurity when they see it used on
others, a sort of feeling that their turn may come, and
so the asylum becomes to them a prison-house and not
a hospital." [2]

Another evil of restraint, even when slight, not always
taken into the consideration it deserves, is that, in
addition to the mental irritation it excites, it acts
injuriously on the health, by its interference with the
ordinary calls of nature, and by the dirty habits it
engenders. A further evil, which is inseparable from
the employment of restraints, is its well-known de-
moralizing effects upon the attendants. Very early

[1] See the effects of putting a patient into a strait-jacket, *Memoir*,
p. 25.
[2] Manning, *op. citat.*, p. 119.

after the adoption of the non-restraint system, its humanizing effect on the character and conduct of the attendants was particularly remarked. Thus in whatever way non-restraint is viewed, its advantages are apparent; while it is just the reverse as regards restraint.

The black spot in the treatment of the insane in America is the sad condition of the lunatics, for whom there is no longer room in the public asylums, and who are consequently confined in workhouses, almshouses, and some of them even in prisons. The disclosures of the treatment to which these poor helpless creatures are subjected, as described by Dr. Willard, is only to be compared with their worst treatment in Europe at the end of last and beginning of the present century.[1]

The Association of Medical Superintendents of American Institutions for the Insane seems admirably conducted, and indeed may be considered itself an institution, and a very useful one. It has existed for upwards of twenty years, and during that period it must have exercised a very beneficial influence upon the members of the Association both professionally and socially; and the circulation of their Reports must also have done much good, by enlightening the public mind on the necessary means for the proper care and treatment of the insane.

[1] See *Notes of a Visit to American Asylums*, by Alexander Robertson, M.D., Physician to the Town's Hospital and City Parochial Asylum, Glasgow : *Journal of Mental Science*, April, 1869.

Among the propositions adopted at the meetings of
the Association, I add an extract of one on the organization of asylums, which might be adopted in this
country with great advantage.

"The physician should be the superintendent and
chief executive officer of the establishment. Besides
being a well-educated physician, he should possess the
mental, physical and social qualities to fit him for the
post. He should serve during good behaviour, reside
on, or very near the premises, and his compensation
should be so liberal as to enable him to devote his
whole time and energies to the welfare of the hospital.
He should nominate to the Board suitable persons to act
as assistant physician, steward and matron; he should
have the entire control of the medical, moral and
dietetic treatment of the patients, the unreserved
power of appointment and discharge of all persons
engaged in their care, and should exercise a general
supervision and direction of every department of the
institution."

"The steward, under the direction of the superintending physician, and by his order, should make all pur-
chases for the institution, keep the accounts, make
engagements with, and pay and discharge those employed about the establishment; have a supervision of
the farm, garden and grounds, and perform such other
duties as may be assigned him."

XIV.

NON-RESTRAINT :—" *La plus haute expression de ce qu'il est possible de réaliser dans l'intérêt de l'amélioration intellectuelle, physique, et morale des aliénés, confiés à nos soins.*"

MOREL, Le Non-restraint, p. 37.

NON-RESTRAINT :—" *A short term to express the absence of all irritation, and to imply the presence of everything that is calculated to soothe the troubled mind into healthfulness and peace.*"

HITCHMAN, Report on Derbyshire Asylum, 1854.

IT is now about thirty years since Dr. Conolly established non-restraint in the treatment of the insane, in the fullest acceptation of the term, in an asylum containing upwards of eight hundred patients, and for the last twenty or twenty-five years that system has been practised in every public asylum in this kingdom. Yet notwithstanding the acknowledged advantages of the system,—its soothing influence upon the insane,— its marked effect in diminishing the violence of the paroxysms of mania,—its tranquillizing effect on the whole inmates of the asylum,—and its beneficial influence on the attendants,—although all this has been witnessed and acknowledged by those who have visited our asylums, the majority of foreign physicians still hesitate to adopt it. It may even be doubted, if in the whole of Europe six asylums could at this time be found beyond Great Britain, where non-restraint is *fully* received and acted on.

But although Dr. Conolly's system of treatment has not been fully or generally adopted out of Great Britain, it has nevertheless exercised a powerful and pervading influence in ameliorating the treatment of the insane, both in Europe and America. It was, indeed, almost impossible that the knowledge of Dr. Conolly's practice, and of its remarkable results on so large a scale in England, could fail to make some impression on the medical superintendents of foreign lunatic establishments, by leading them to contrast their treatment with that adopted in England, first at Hanwell, and afterwards throughout the whole kingdom. Good was done in this way, but not so much as might have been expected : there is now, however, the prospect of a brighter future for the treatment of the lunatic in Continental countries. Some of the most distinguished foreign physicians have not only accepted non-restraint, but have become earnest and eloquent advocates of the system in its entirety. Dr. Morel in France, Professor Griesinger[1] and Dr. Ludwig Meyer in Germany, Dr. Ewarts in

[1] When this sheet was in the hands of the publisher, the melancholy account of Professor Griesinger's death reached us. By the death of this distinguished physician, psychological science has lost one of its ablest interpreters, and the insane one of their most earnest and enlightened friends. He died 26th of October of iliac abscess, at the early age of 51.

Holland, Dr. Tebaldi in Italy, and Dr. Ernst Salomon in Sweden, completely satisfied themselves by personal observation of the great advantage of treating the insane without the use of mechanical restraint. And the forcible language in which these physicians have expressed their conviction of the benefits from such a mode of treatment, will, it is hoped, make many converts, and lead soon to an adoption of the system, in their respective countries, as universally as in Britain.

It has been sometimes objected that it cannot be a sound principle to adopt non-restraint in the treatment of the insane, as an absolute and inflexible law. The answer is, that it has not been so adopted. When properly stated, the principle is this—that mechanical restraint should never be resorted to, unless there be a clear necessity, and that the existence of the clear necessity should not be too readily accepted. With many physicians this ends in finding the cases, in which restraint is deemed necessary, to be so rare as practically not to exist: they do not positively abolish restraint, they simply never use it, because they never deem it necessary. They regard it as in the highest degree desirable to avoid it, from considerations both of humanity and science; and having adopted this view, they find that it is not needed in cases in which it would probably be employed by physicians less strongly impressed with the desirability of avoiding it, and therefore less anxious to discover a substitute, in methods of treatment which are more humane, and

in better accord with the teachings of physiology
and psychology. Even those who defend the use of
restraint in certain cases, are nearly always careful to
point out that they find the number of such cases to
be small, and their pride is in the largeness of the
number of the non-restrained. The soundness of the
principle of non-restraint is thus often acknowledged,
even in the defence of restraint ; and perhaps further
and more earnest efforts might make the small number
still smaller, till at length the list of the restrained
would be a blank.

It is desirable, therefore, that it should be understood
that there is no such thing as an absolute repudiation
of restraint in the treatment of the insane. The
warmest advocates of non-restraint admit that cases
may occur in which it is proper to resort to mechanical
restraint, and by this admission we do not think that
we invalidate the principle, which is not of universal
application, though it is made as nearly universal as
possible, and is departed from only when the necessity
for doing so is clear, and then with a regret that there
is no better way of attaining the object.

With the view of ascertaining how often, and for
what reasons, it is found necessary in practice to de-
viate from a strict adherence to the non-restraint system, and whether seclusion or active exercise in the
open air is considered and employed as a substitute
for restraint, I applied to some of the senior medical
superintendents of our large asylums for the results
of their experience on the subject. What follows is the

result of this enquiry, and it shows that, while the non-restraint system is not carried out in this country as an *inflexible* rule, it is found necessary to have recourse to restraint so rarely, and then under such exceptional circumstances, as to amount practically to a total disappearance of restraint in the treatment of insanity.

Dr. Campbell, of the Essex County Asylum, containing 599 patients, replies that since the establishment of the Asylum in 1853, during which time 2568 patients have been under his treatment, on one occasion only did he find it necessary to restrain a violent, destructive male patient for four hours by a strait-jacket, which he had to procure for the purpose.

Dr. Mackintosh, of the Royal Asylum, Glasgow, with 605 patients, states that he has not employed mechanical restraint for the last twenty years, and that seclusion is very little used,—active exercise being found a good substitute.

Dr. Thurnam, the Medical Superintendent of the Wilts County Asylum, with 450 patients, since 1851, says that mechanical restraint has not been employed during that time, except in two or three surgical cases, to retain bandages ; that seclusion is rarely used ; that months often elapse without a single instance of seclusion ; and that active exercise in the open air is found very beneficial in cases when seclusion would otherwise be employed.

Dr. Palmer, of the Lincoln Asylum, with 562 patients, says that since 1852, when the Asylum was opened, no mechanical restraint has been employed

M

in it; that seclusion for short periods in the ordinary bedrooms is occasionally resorted to.

Dr. Hitchman, of the Derby County Asylum, with 335 patients, who began to practice non-restraint in 1842 in a private asylum, and was subsequently medical officer at Hanwell for five years, states that he never had occasion to use restraint in the Derbyshire Asylum, till last year, when in a case of hysterical mania in a young woman, who was bent on plucking out her tongue, he placed the hands of the patient in gloves, too large to be put into the mouth. This is the only instance he says, out of 2796 lunatics treated, in which he has found it necessary to have recourse to restraint.

Dr. T. Jones, for 21 years the Medical Superintendent of the North Wales Counties' Lunatic Asylum, with 371 patients, says that he has never had occasion to use mechanical restraint in any shape, and that seclusion is only resorted to in extreme cases, and then for as short a time as possible,—slighter cases in their own rooms, and violent epileptic cases in a padded room. Active exercise in the open air, when practicable, he adds, is always preferred to seclusion.

Dr. John Kirkman, of the Suffolk County Asylum, with 416 patients, says that he has not used mechanical restraint since 1831; that he rarely employs seclusion, and that active exercise is substituted for it with the best results.

Mr. Broadhurst, Superintendent of the Lancaster Asylum for 20 years, with a number of patients ranging from 700 to 1000, says:—" During the whole of that period, I have not put any patient under mechanical restraint, nor have I seen a case in which I thought that the use of it would have been beneficial.

"Seclusion, as a means of treatment, must often be needed in cases of acute mania, with a tendency to violence. In epilepsy, seclusion is also a valuable remedy. The padded room is only required for those who have lost all control over their movements. We have daily proofs of the advantage of active exercise in other ways, than as a substitute for seclusion."

It appears from these Reports, that considerable reliance is placed by physicians of long experience in the treatment of the insane on the value of active exercise in the open air as a substitute for seclusion. In addition to the foregoing testimony on this subject, I may state that Dr. Howden, of the Montrose Royal Asylum, with about 400 inmates, has not had a patient either in seclusion or under restraint for six years. He attaches great importance to out-door exercise as a part of general treatment.

But to enable physicians satisfactorily to adopt non-restraint, Governments have an important duty to perform. The existing asylums in many parts of Europe, are often ill-adapted for the proper care and treatment of the insane, for which purpose, indeed, a considerable proportion of them were not originally intended. Such establishments must be replaced by suitable buildings, so as to give the physicians in charge of them facilities for the proper treatment of their

M 2

patients. To do this effectually is an imperative duty of the Governments, under whose rule such unsuitable asylums exist; and the nations which neglect to fulfil so high a duty, after they are made acquainted with the miserable condition of their insane, incur a heavy responsibility, and place themselves in the rear of civilization.[1]

Dr. Conolly remarks that—"The difficulties attending the introduction of the non-restraint system into properly constructed and appointed asylums, have been greatly exaggerated by those who have been habituated only to the use of coercion in attempts to subdue the violent or obstinate lunatic, and who have never thought of any other mode of treatment." The superintendent of an Italian asylum is reported to have said to an English physician, that *the notion of keeping several hundred lunatics in one house, without ever having recourse to restraint was the most preposterous thing he ever heard of*—and yet Dr. Conolly, in less than four months, accomplished *this preposterous thing*, in a house containing upwards of eight hundred lunatics. The following is his own account of this feat. It will be remembered that he took charge of Hanwell Asylum on the 1st of June.

"After the *first* of July, when I required a daily return to be made to me of the number of patients restrained, there were never more than eighteen so treated on one day, a number that would seem reason-

---

[1] *See Appendix A. for further information on this subject.*

ably small out of 800 patients, but for the fact that after the *thirty-first* of July, the number so confined never exceeded *eight;* and after the *twelfth* of August never exceeded *one;* and that after the *twentieth* of September no restraints were employed at all." [1]

"It is scarcely possible," Dr. Conolly adds, "to convey by words the various ways in which the difficulties (the mere imagination of which alarms those not familiar with the insane), vanish before the patience, firmness, and ingenuity of officers who are determined that no difficulties in accomplishing their object, shall be regarded as insuperable."

"One general error," he also observes, "seems to pervade the minds of those who most readily condemn the abolition of restraints; they always assume that if one kind of restraint is discontinued, some other kind of restraint must be substituted for it." Dr. Morel makes a like remark :—"Une chose préoccupe encore les médecins aliénistes Français, et cela ressort de toutes les lettres que j'ai reçues—c'est la substitution d'un moyen de contrainte à un autre." [2]

In order to understand the practical application of the non-restraint treatment, in such a way as to enable physicians to adopt it with confidence, Dr. Conolly considered it very desirable that they should witness its operation in an asylum in which it is fully carried out, and where the whole arrangements of the institution may be regarded as intimately associated with, and

[1] *Treatment of the Insane*, p. 179.　　[2] *Op. citat.*, p. 72.

forming the complement of, the non-restraint system. "The mere abolition of fetters and mechanical restraints constitutes only a part of what is properly called the non-restraint system. Its influence pervades the whole institution, affects the character of every act, and the conduct of every person in the asylum." [1]

Foreign physicians who, acting on this suggestion, visit England, may feel certain of a cordial reception from the medical superintendents of our asylums, and of obtaining every facility in making their enquiries, for which sufficient time should be allowed.

Dr. Morel's description of the manner in which he himself examined the practice of non-restraint, and the whole management of our asylums, is so excellent, that I take the liberty of quoting it, and recommending it as an example to be followed by other physicians in their enquiries:—

"Je ne me suis pas contenté, en effet, de visiter en passant les asiles Anglais; j'y ai séjourné, j'y ai vécu de la vie des médecins et je pourrais presque dire de l'existence des infirmiers et des malades. Aucun détail de cette vie intime du jour, de la nuit, de tous les instants, ne m'a échappé. Je pouvais, à toute heure et isolément, aller et venir, m'entretenir avec les aliénés, voir de près comment ils étaient soignés et traités; j'étais, en un mot, aussi libre dans mes mouvements, aussi peu gêné dans mes appréciations, qu'il m'est donné de l'être à l'asile de Saint Yon." [2]

[1] *Treatment of the Insane*, p. 35.   [2] *Op. citat.*, p. 20.

XV.

Dr. Conolly's labours began to tell upon his health during the progress of the introduction of the non-restraint system into Hanwell Asylum, and he was obliged in the midst of it to retire for a short time to the country for rest. The following fragment is extracted from a letter written at this time to his friend Mr. W. Savage Landor, and kindly sent to me by Mr. Foster. " There is a stanza," he writes, " in a certain Ode to Robert Southey, which I repeat almost daily, beginning, ' We hurry to the river we must cross,' and it always consoles me, and renews my wish not to let the mind languish as years advance upon me, but rather, following the author's inspiring example, to continue thinking and doing, to the last, such worthy things as may take away all dreariness from that inevitable stream." (Aug. 31, 1849.)

This note, so characteristic of Conolly's mind, was written when he had just established non-restraint in Hanwell Asylum, and when he had doubtless begun to feel the influence of ten years' anxious work on a constitution never very robust. He saw that he had still much work before him, and he resolved to meet it.

When Dr. Conolly ceased to be Resident Physician,

the office was not continued, and he was appointed
Visiting Physician. From this time he entered on a
large practice, which, with asylum duties that he still
retained, began in a few years to affect his health. He
suffered at times from chronic rheumatism, complicated
with neuralgic pains, and an irritable state of the
skin. His general health also began to fail, and his
capacity for mental work gradually diminished; he
felt, he said, that age was creeping upon him, and,
under this feeling, he gradually withdrew from practice, and wisely retired to his country residence, Lawn
House, near the scene of his most important labours.
His time in Lawn House was not, however, passed in
inactivity. In the early part of his retirement, and
before his strength had failed so much that his powers
of mind ceased to obey his summons, he published in
the medical journals some excellent commentaries on
the Insanity of Children; and papers on the Phy-
siognomy of Insanity, and on other subjects relating
to lunacy. He continued to be consulted in difficult
cases, and had a large and anxious professional correspondence till within a few years of his death. The following extracts from his letters show how gradually he
lost power, and how conscious he was of the loss, and
how calmly he bore it.

The early failure of Dr. Conolly's health and mental
energy is greatly to be lamented, as we have most
probably lost some useful matter on the nature and
treatment of insanity. In a letter to his friend, M.
Battel, dated 1858, he writes: " I wish much to review

my notes of cases in my private practice of the last twenty years, and to leave, although not in a systematic form, some useful commentaries; but perhaps this is only the last deceptious dream of life." It proved to be but the day dream of an exhausted mind; although Dr. Conolly lived five years after writing this letter to his friend, his mental energy was never sufficiently restored to enable him to commence his proposed work.

The following extracts from a letter also addressed to M. Battel, a few years later (May 1862), shows his gradually increasing weakness, accompanied with a depressing feeling of sadness: "It seems long since I had the happiness of receiving one of your friendly and charming letters. To hear from you again, and to be assured that you are well, will be a real consolation to me. I am conscious on my own part, that I ought to have said this long ago, and my excuse must be, in part, that in the last two years, the cheerfulness which would have prompted me to write to you, has sustained many assaults, which, although they have not overcome me, have often saddened me, and caused me to refrain from troubling my esteemed friends with my thoughts. And amongst these friends, be assured, my dear Monsieur Battel, you hold a high place, and will always do so whilst I remain among the living. The year 1861, and the commencement of the present year, have deprived me of *many* friends known to me from my earliest days. One of the last died in April; and a dear daughter of Dr. and Mrs. Tuke died, after a short illness, soon afterward. This last event caused me

especial grief, for I loved the dear child extremely.
The next morning it would appear that I had an attack
of cerebral congestion, which made me insensible for
some hours. Happily it left no paralysis, and no mental
disorder, but I feel weak, and indisposed to any long-
continued mental exertion. I am now resuming my
ordinary occupations, but to say the truth, with some
feeling of regret. After a few weeks of tranquillity, I
feel unwilling to return into the world, which has now
very few attractions for me.

"Whenever I am ill and tranquil, I have a singular
pleasure, as I must have told you before, in reading
French. The language is associated in my mind with
the early days of my life and my earliest studies. For
the last few weeks I have delighted to look again at an
old copy of the 'Lettres de Messire Roger de Rabutin,
Comte de Bussy,' &c.; and from these I have turned
to a much prized book, given to me by your good self,
the 'Memoirs, &c., &c., of the Marquise de Sévigné,' by
Walckenaer, in which I only find one fault, that I go on
reading it too long, unwilling to close the book. Finding in one volume an account of Mme. de Sévigné's
journey down the Loire, I was enchanted to read a
description of some localities on the borders of the
Loire which were once familiar to me. Mont Louis and
Veretz, near Tours, I remember well; and the expressions of praise in the letters seem to me not exaggerated: 'le pays est le plus charmant qu'aucun autre
qui soit sur la terre habitable.' The cottage in which
I lived in 1818 is beautifully situated on the right

bank of the Loire, opposite Tours, and has acquired subsequent celebrity as the residence for a time of Béranger. It is called the Grénadière, and a pomegranate tree grew over the front of it. Of that agreeable cottage I have some descriptions written on the spot. I shall, however, content myself by referring you to the 'Dernières Chansons de P. J. de Béranger,' p. 103, 'Les Oiseaux de la Grénadière.' But I must suspend these retrospections of an invalid, relying on your indulgence. I shall be impatient to hear that you are well, and you will tell me also of the health of M. Falret, whom we both much esteem."

The following letter is a reply to the author of this Memoir, who had suggested to Dr. Conolly to write his views more fully than he had hitherto done on the Insanity of old age :—

" Dec. 8, 1862. I have been meaning every day to acknowledge your most kind letter of the 29th ult., but I fear I must myself be feeling one of the diseases of age invading me ; for I have days of languor now and then, which, when the day is gone, make me unable to account for how it has been spent. It is rather curious that the subject of the Delusions of old age, concerning which you enquire if I have written anything, has been lately and often the particular subject of my thoughts. For many years past I have kept rather full records of cases occurring in my practice, and I have got a sort of alphabetical list of them ; but to consider them in various classes—as insanity in children, and at the age of puberty, and in middle age, and in decline, &c.—

seems a task I can hardly hope to accomplish. The *children's* cases were despatched in a few papers called ' Recollections,' in the ' Medical Times,' early this year; but then came an illness, I fear a temporary congestion of the brain, in April, and I have not thought it prudent since to write for the press. Now, however, I hope to go on, although very cautiously, and my next papers will be on the subject of Senile Insanity. I have some curious cases, and your remarks will not be lost upon me. It is too evident that the brain loses its general energy as the body does; but it seems as if certain portions of it decline differently in different persons, and the action of other portions becomes uncontrolled. Forgetfulness of words, of dates, of people, of things read and things once carefully done or written; dread of poverty; visions of wealth; foolish attachments, and dislikes; strange delusions, founded on dreams; and sometimes the oddest singularities. These things are very curious, and Phrenology, which seems forgotten, appears the only doctrine that tends to explain them.

" Perhaps the wonder is that any of us retain cheerfulness, for the loss of our friends is inevitable and dreadful, and whatever we do or think of, the hopes that cheered us no longer animate us to exertion. It is still a great blessing to retain one's *mind*, and to feel tranquilly assured that whatever has happened, and whatever is to follow, has been and will be regulated by a First Cause—all wise and all good. In our profound darkness as to the kind of existence that will follow this brief and transitory state, the hope and belief that our best affections will form its happiness seem inherent, and as it were instinctive in us. Our great Creator surely did not implant these hopes in us to mock us. Certainly as we approach the end of this mortal life we feel more and more that we are gradually becoming quite detached from it. The body slowly perishes and will not *let* the mind act freely, but the consciousness that the mind is *still* living, and capable of living, seems never to fade."

The subjoined extract, from another letter to the author of this memoir, was written a few weeks only before Dr. Conolly left Lawn House (Dec. 1865). Its subdued melancholy tone showed that he then had the impression that his end was near at hand: "I am ashamed to see the date of your most kind letter (Oct. 14) not acknowledged. The part of it relative to your own good health, and of your rational life, away from crowds, gratified me more than I can express. Your kind enquiries as to my own state and mode of living reminded me of many things dear to my memory. Since my paralytic warnings a year and a half since, although I have no paralysis, I *feel* that all my energies decline. I am sure I could write something about the creeping on of old age truer than what Cicero wrote, for the *De Senectute* was composed when he was *only* 63, and I am 71. It is, however, a great blessing to retain one's rational faculties, and to be perfectly content and grateful to the AUTHOR of our being, on whom we all depend. I shall in a few weeks hear the birds of the Lawn no more, and shall no more

see the trees familiar to me, nor the old Asylum still
within view. But the recollections of scenes in *that*
building will gladden my heart as long as I live ; recollections so precious, that I often say I ought to be
content with them, if every other blessing had been
withheld from me."

The vicinity of Lawn House to Hanwell was evidently
a source of great and abiding pleasure to Dr. Conolly.
Even when writing his last work, *The Treatment of
the Insane*, he breaks out in the following apostrophe
on the " old Asylum," showing with what satisfaction his
mind dwelt on the benefit conferred, chiefly by his own
labours, on its " crazy children."

" No longer residing in the Hanwell Asylum, and no
longer superintending it, or even visiting it, I continue
to live within view of the building, and its familiar trees
and grounds. The sound of the bell that announces
the hour of the patients' dinner still gives me pleasure,
because I know that it summons the poorest creature
there to a comfortable, well-prepared, and sufficient
meal ; and the tone of the chapel bell, coming across
the narrow valley of the Brent, still reminds me, morning and evening, of the well remembered and mingled
congregation of the afflicted, and who are then assem-
bling, humble, yet hopeful and not forgotten, and not
spiritually deserted."

From this time (December, 1865) Dr. Conolly continued much in the same state, although gradually
becoming more feeble ; but his mind remained clear
and tranquil, and his interest in everything connected

with what had been the labour of his life remained
unabated. In this state he had an attack of paralysis
accompanied with convulsions, which proved fatal in
a few hours, March 5, 1867.

Thus passed away a good man, having fairly earned
a reputation as a practical philanthropist, which will
carry his name down to posterity among the benefactors
of his race.

If the state of a man's mind during the last years of
his life discloses the feelings with which he looks back
on the part he has played in the position allotted
to him, then Dr. Conolly's retrospect must have been
very satisfactory. He exhibited during the period of
his retirement a tranquil, contented, and happy state of
mind; and he doubtless enjoyed the consolation of feeling that his life had been one of active benevolence,
and that his labours had contributed largely to the
permanent alleviation of human suffering in the "most
calamitous of all diseases."

XVI.

THE failure of mental energy which Dr. Conolly experienced, and to which he refers on various occasions
in his correspondence, as gradually creeping on him, is
felt by all who reach an advanced age, and by some at
a comparatively early period of life.   In the former, the
failure is generally the consequence of the natural
decay of the system in which the brain participates.
In the latter it is often the result of over mental work,
inducing premature cerebral exhaustion, and may occur
at very different ages,—earlier generally in proportion
to the amount and character of the mental work, and
the delicacy of the individual constitution.

It is to the latter class of cases, those namely in
which there occurs a failure of mental power not due to
age, that the following observations chiefly apply.   The
subject is one little understood by the public, and it
has scarcely I think, received the attention of medical
writers, to which it is entitled by its importance.

Failure of the power for mental work may attract
little notice for a time, and even when observed it
may not be attributed to the real cause, but rather to
dyspepsia, or some derangement of the general health.
The symptoms of the condition here alluded to vary in

different cases. One of the earliest, Dr. Conolly mentions, is lassitude, with disinclination for mental work. Headache is a very common symptom, especially towards the end of the day's work; and this is generally a dull, rather than an acute pain, with a sense of exhaustion and inability to exert the mind. Giddiness is not unusual. The nights are frequently passed in wakefulness, or the sleep is unrefreshing, and there is often drowsiness during the day. Impairment or confusion of memory then becomes apparent, with an inability to concentrate the attention on a subject for any length of time, or to unravel questions which some time before would have required little effort. Proneness to irritability is also often observed, while in other cases, the tendency is to mental depression. When this last is a marked symptom, it should always be regarded as serious.

If work is still persevered in, under such indications of cerebral exhaustion, general derangement of the mental faculties may ensue. " There can be no greater error," Dr. Conolly remarks, " than at any period of life to urge the failing mental powers to a state of complete exhaustion; derangement of the whole mental faculties may be the consequence."

When there exists any hereditary tendency to insanity, the risks are greatly increased; and young persons of a delicate constitution and sensitive nervous system cannot in general bear severe or long-continued mental work, especially if attended with anxiety.

The subjoined case, which occurred to myself in the

N

early part of my practice in London, is given to show in how short a time severe and exciting mental work may induce complete mental derangement. A young man, a member of Parliament, in office at the time, undertook the preparation of a Government Bill of some intricacy. He laboured incessantly for, I believe, many weeks at the preparation of the Bill, often at night as well as by day. The Bill was well received by the House, and he was complimented on his success. It was remarked however by some of the members that he appeared excited during the course of the evening when the measure was introduced. The effect of his success was more than his exhausted brain could bear. The following morning he got up in a greatly excited state, affirming that he had just been ordered to proceed on an important mission to Spain, and was full of preparations for his immediate departure. It was all a delusion, and he continued insane, and died a few years afterwards.

Anxiety about the success of the Bill,—a condition which greatly increased the danger arising from the prolonged and severe mental work,—told in the case of this gentleman on a rather delicate constitution. Still, had the labour been extended over a longer period, and confined to day work, though the brain might have been fatigued, rest for a time would probably have restored it to its normal state, and the distressing result might thus have been averted. This is the lesson to be learned from the case.

When the brain has been called on to do work

beyond its powers, it never fails to give signs of exhaustion, sooner or later; and at whatever age these occur, or whatever form they assume, they should be treated as warnings that must not be neglected.   They show that the organ of the mind is unable to sustain the efforts to which it has been, or is still being subjected, and that it requires rest.

The obvious remedy in these cases is cessation, more or less complete, from work.   In the slighter cases, when the indications of failing power have been early attended to, and their cause understood, a reduction of the amount of work, with attention to the general health, may be sufficient to restore the normal energy of the nervous system; but in the more serious cases, total abstinence from all mental work will generally be necessary, for a period commensurate with the degree of exhaustion, and the constitution of the individual. Along with this, of course, effective measures for the restoration of the general health which, in such cases, always suffers, must be adopted.   And when the general health and mental energy appear to be restored, the amount of work which experience has shown the brain to be unequal to, must not be resumed.   By adopting these measures in good time, valuable lives may be prolonged in the possession of a large share of restored health, and in the enjoyment of mental powers still capable of much useful work—provided always that the amount be proportioned to that of the restored mental energy. The period given to recovery, however, should never be too strictly limited.   " The danger in these cases,"

Dr. Conolly well observes, "arises from a return to active mental work after partial recovery."

In some cases where the exhaustion has been very great, it may be necessary to abstain permanently from a return to the work which produced the evil; but in other cases the resumption of this work to a moderate amount is allowable, and may be beneficial, since a *total and prolonged* cessation from the exercise of the mind on subjects to which it has been long habituated may tend to impede the return of its normal vigour. In such cases, however, the work should not be resumed till the brain has had sufficient rest, and has given clear indications of returning power; and even then, it should be resumed gradually, and to such an extent only as shall incur no risk of inducing a relapse. One of the most important rules, on resuming mental work, is to restrict it to *short* periods at a time, to be increased only as the sense of restored mental energy is experienced, and never till a feeling of exhaustion is induced.

In all persons, after a certain age, which however varies in different constitutions, a reduction of active mental work is wise, and tends to secure the preservation of mental vigour. But even in advanced years a moderate exercise of the mind, especially on subjects which are familiar and still interesting, is beneficial, as a means of maintaining the integrity of the brain, and of continuing the possession of the mental powers, till they fade naturally with the decline of life. This careful regulation of work may in some instances avert those singular and often painful exhibitions of mental weakness or aberration which are classed under *senile insanity*, and which are often a cause of distress to the relatives of the sufferer.

It does not come within the scope of these observations to notice the changes in the brain itself which result from excessive mental work. The object is rather to indicate the signs by which we may know that the organ is being overtasked, and to urge the application of the proper remedy, before structural change of the brain has occurred.

Little, indeed, is known of the changes which occur in the incipient stage; but as Dr. Conolly remarks,— " However ignorant we may be of the primary changes in the brain by over exertion of its functions, we may at least gather wisdom from a consideration of their undoubted results." The primary changes induced in the brain by overwork, may elude our observation, but the consequences of perseverance in such work after due warnings, leave no doubt that structural disease of the brain is in many cases eventually the result.

Instances may occur to the reader of these remarks, of persons whose brains have been actively at work through the whole of a long life, and who still continue to show more mental energy and power than is usual in advanced years. Such instances, however, are to be regarded as exceptions. They are generally found in men of robust constitutions, who have been chiefly occupied in pursuits attended with little anxiety, or

who have had the finer emotions and feelings habitually
under control. It deserves also to be borne in mind,
that these rare and exceptional cases are apt to become
the objects of general observation and remark, while
the many, the vigour of whose mental powers has been
shortened by excessive work, disappear without notice,
and too often, even without the cause of their early
decline being rightly understood.

Let it not, however, be imagined that either the
subject or author of this Memoir wish to discourage the
active employment of the mental faculties. It is known
to all who are acquainted with the physiological laws
by which health and growth are regulated, that exercise of the brain is as necessary to insure the health
and full development of the mental faculties, as is exercise of the limbs to insure the vigour and full development of the muscular system. But there is a limit to
the extent to which these exercises should be carried.
If overdone, the object may be frustrated. To obtain
their full benefit they must be suited, both as regards
muscle and brain, to the age and constitution of the
individual, and should never be pushed to excess.
There is no greater danger to the future intellectual
prospects of talented children, particularly of those
giving indications of precocious mental endowments,
than the injudicious management of their early education. The early chapters of Dr. Conolly's work on the
Indications of Insanity, and his papers on *Infantile
Insanity*, contain much sound and valuable advice on
this subject. He very judiciously urges the necessity

of strict attention to the general health as the best
means of insuring and maintaining the full action of
the mental powers. In forcing the education of talented
children, he points out that a grave error is often committed. Such children are generally of a susceptible
nervous constitution, and ought to be restrained rather
than encouraged to learn, till they acquire a healthy
physical development, and reach an age sufficient to
warrant active mental exertion. Until that time has
arrived, they should, if possible, reside in the country,
and have good, plain, wholesome food, with abundant
and joyous exercise in the open air to insure their
physical health; and their mental education should be
limited chiefly to the cultivation of their observing
faculties—their attention being directed to the natural
objects surrounding them. By such a training and
mode of life, many talented children, who have delicate
constitutions, might lay the foundation of future mental
and bodily health, so as to eventually attain the eminence of which their early talents gave promise. Instances of the injurious effects of over mental work at
a later period of youth are occasionally observed among
the students in our Universities, who, in the struggle
for honours or distinction, endeavour to acquire in a
few months an amount of knowledge, in the acquisition
of which, many months, or even years, ought to have
been spent. In delicate constitutions such a strain
may have the effect of diminishing the mental energy
for the remainder of life.

XVII.

DR. CONOLLY was a man of great natural talents, and possessed a highly cultivated mind: his views on all subjects of social economy were liberal and enlightened, and he took an active part in the various movements which have of late years been directed to the amelioration and improvement of the poorer classes. In social life he was much esteemed for his kind and amiable disposition and cheerful manner: he was a most agreeable companion, whom it was always a pleasure to meet. He was held in great respect by his profession generally, and for many years had a large consulting practice in his own department; indeed he was long the chief consulting physician in this country in difficult cases of insanity and of other diseases of the nervous system. His opinion was especially sought after in the more important cases *de lunatico inquirendo,*—his evidence being always given clearly and forcibly, and the verdict of the jury almost invariably in unison with it. He was much dissatisfied with our mode of dealing with such cases; he thought it an unsatisfactory and improper thing to determine the soundness or unsoundness of a person's mind by the opinion of an ordinary jury. He also strongly condemned the system of medical witnesses being engaged, not to give an independent opinion of the case, but one in accordance with the interest of the party by whom they are employed. Such a practice he justly stigmatised as derogatory to the character of the profession and injurious to the public.[1]

The University of Oxford conferred on Dr. Conolly the honorary degree of D.C.L., and in foreign countries he was well known and greatly honoured for his unceasing exertions in the cause of the insane.

It might have been naturally expected that, from his large consulting practice in cases of insanity and diseases of the nervous system generally, and the extent to which his opinion was sought in medico-legal questions, that Dr. Conolly would have died rich. It was far otherwise, however; and this may be chiefly explained by his professional position, during the greater part of his life,—a physician in small country towns, and afterwards as Resident Physician in the Hanwell Asylum, when his income was barely sufficient to maintain his family. He was also very liberal-minded in his practice and otherwise, and gave little attention to financial matters. Still he had sufficient to supply all his wants during his retirement, and to leave something to his family at his death.

He left a son and three daughters; one of his daughters being married to a clergyman, and two to eminent psychological physicians.

---

[1] The legal method of deciding such cases in France, under the Code Napoleon, is more in accordance with medical science and the dictates of common sense.

Although, as will be noticed in a future part of this Memoir, Dr. Conolly took a warm and often an active interest in the progress of medical and general science, the great object of his life was to increase our knowledge of insanity, to improve the treatment of the insane, and, above all, to demonstrate the benefits of non-restraint.

Without the least desire to detract from the well-earned and acknowledged merits of Dr. Charlesworth and Mr. Gardiner Hill as the first to introduce the non-restraint treatment, and without questioning the encouragement and assistance which their example afforded to Dr. Conolly (always cordially acknowledged by him), I think no one who reads the account of his labours in Hanwell Asylum, given in these pages, can doubt that he would have introduced non-restraint into that institution had he never heard of what had been done in Lincoln.

Dr. Conolly's attention was first directed to the subject of Insanity on visiting a lunatic asylum in Glasgow when a boy; the impression made on his mind by that visit seems never to have been effaced, and it was deepened some years afterwards by his perusal of the works of Pinel and William Tuke. He had acquired a sufficient knowledge of mental disease to make it the subject of his inaugural dissertation on taking his medical degree in the University of Edinburgh, when about twenty-six years old.

From this time his thoughts seem to have been much

occupied in meditating on the treatment of the insane, and his friend Dr. Thomson, of Leamington, told me that, when he was practising at Stratford, he was so anxious to have charge of a lunatic asylum that he had the thoughts of establishing one himself, and we have already been told of his great desire to become Physician to the Hanwell Asylum when it was first established. This desire was happily accomplished, and we have seen that by his successful efforts in that asylum, he not only placed non-restraint on a permanent basis, but, as has been elegantly expressed, "he expounded the humane and scientific theory of it, and set forth eloquently the wide, reaching, and beneficial consequences of its adoption. He not only made the hitherto obscure movement a world-known success, but he made reaction impossible. Justly, therefore, is his name associated with this noble work of progress; his life justly identified with this glorious chapter of human development." [1]

On the value of Dr. Conolly's successful efforts in the cause of the insane, Sir Thomas Watson, Bart., President of the Royal College of Physicians of London, in his obituary notice thus expresses himself:—

"Dr. Conolly's renown will rest, and his name will go down to a late posterity, upon his having been the first and foremost in redressing and abolishing that hideous neglect, those cruel methods of restraint and even torture, which had been the scandal of our land, in

---

[1] *Obituary Memoir of Dr. Conolly*, by Dr. Maudsley: *Journal of Mental Science*, July, 1866.

respect of the treatment of the insane. He showed, not merely by eloquent and pathetic reasoning, but by the testimony of undeniable facts, that most of the shackles and privations which had been imposed upon those unhappy beings were unnecessary and hurtful, and that their release from needless bodily misery and degradation tended more than any other thing to restore, or, when restoration was impossible, to improve, their mental health. The spirit of John Conolly was congenial with the spirit of John Howard; and their noble example has left behind them, and encouraged, a similar spirit, which is actively and widely at work in this nation."

Nor was Dr. Conolly's fame confined to his own country. The late Professor Guislain, of Belgium, one of the most distinguished alienist physicians in Europe, says of him: "Posterity will hold the name of Conolly in grateful remembrance for the annihilating condemnation which he hurled against the agents of coercion." [1]

At the annual meeting of the Medico-Psychological Association, of which Dr. Conolly had been twice president, held in Edinburgh, Dr. W. A. F. Browne, Commissioner in Lunacy for Scotland, who long enjoyed the friendship of Dr. Conolly, thus spoke of him in his presidential address :—

"John Conolly displayed, within the University of this town, and in the arena of the Royal Medical Society— dear to many of those who hear me—those predilections and preferences which ultimately determined his destiny,

[1] *Leçons Orales*, tom. iii. p. 181.

and gave him a position of nearly equal rank among
physicians and philanthropists. His thesis was on
Insanity, and formed the foundation of that work by
which he is most popularly known. A physician in
increasing practice, one of the editors and originators
of the *British and Foreign Medical Review and Clyclo-
pædia of Practical Medicine*, and a teacher in a University, John Conolly, I know, never felt that he had
secured his true position, or that he had found a fair
field for the exercise of his head and heart, until he was
appointed Medical Superintendent of Hanwell. It is not
affirmed that he made personal sacrifices in order to
accept this distinction; but, like that of many other
great and good men, his life was one of much sacrifice
and much suffering. It is not my province here, however much it may be my inclination, to speak of more
of his good deeds than of the assistance he offered in
the grand revolution effected in the management, and
of the effects of his teaching in the propagation of sound
views in the treatment of the insane and of the idiotic.
I cannot refrain from claiming him as an advocate—
and as a philosophical advocate—of a medico-psycho-
logy founded upon induction. His ideas, it is true,
seemed to have passed through his heart, and his feelings to have raised and rarefied his intellect. Perhaps
it is because of the elegance and popular attractions of
his style that his habits of thinking have been regarded
as less logical than illustrative; but his *Indications of
Insanity* show a familiarity with the laws of the human
mind, and especially with the peculiarities and subtle

defects by which it is disturbed and unhinged, requiring
great perspicacity and penetration, as well as careful
analysis.

" Sensitive in his rectitude, gentle and genial, he was
to all men conciliating and courteous ; to his friends,
and I judge after an experience of thirty years, he was
almost chivalrously faithful and generous ; and the
insane he positively loved."

At the meeting, at which Dr. Browne pronounced
this elegant and just encomium on his late friend, a
resolution was passed to open a subscription, under the
auspices of the members of the Association, to establish
an annual prize for an essay on Psychology, or some
other fitting memorial of Dr. Conolly ; and Baron
Mundy presented the Association with a marble bust
of the Doctor, executed by the celebrated Roman sculp-
tor, Cav. Benzoni.[1]

At the request of the Association, and by the consent
of the President and Fellows, the bust now finds an
appropriate place in the Royal College of Physicians of
London.   It was presented by Dr. Mundy himself, who
was introduced by Drs. Tuke and Maudsley, the sons-
in-law of Dr. Conolly, the President of the Association

---

[1] Baron Mundy, a German physician, and one of Dr. Conolly's
most esteemed foreign friends, had devoted much time in studying
the nature and treatment of insanity, and had witnessed the treatment in the Hanwell Asylum.   No one appreciated more fully the
value of Dr. Conolly's labours, or exerted himself more strenuously
to diffuse a knowledge of them on the Continent, and to impress
upon the physicians of lunatic asylums the great advantage of the
mild and non-restraint system of treatment.

being unavoidably absent. On presenting the bust
Baron Mundy spoke as follows :—

"Sir Thomas Watson and Gentlemen,—I was highly
gratified at the acceptance of my humble present by my
fellow associates, and likewise proud of the place proposed by the Medico-Psychological Association for it,
subject to your kind assent. I feel myself greatly
honoured in standing to-day before you as one of the
delegates entrusted with the offer of this token. It is
certainly neither here in this place, nor now, that I am
permitted to eulogise a man who will live in the recollection of posterity. But allow me, before I retire, to
allude on this occasion to a passage in your oration of
last year, in which you, after the eloquent tribute paid
to our lamented friend, censure, so justly and ener-
getically, the system of torture practised before the time
of Conolly even in your own country. You have been
enjoying for almost a quarter of a century the work of
the great man who is no more ; and still your neighbours, close to your own shores, have yet, at the moment
I address you, two thousand unfortunate beings tied in
strait-jackets ; and the total number of insane on the
continent confined in cells, fastened in beds, and
strapped up in strait-jackets, amounts in 1867 to fifty
thousand. It is for me, as a foreigner, a humiliation,
and perhaps at the same time a proof of my professional
courage, that I denounce these facts before so high an
authority as yourself, and on so solemn an occasion as
this of to-day. But my aim is only to impress on you
the importance of your continuing to censure this bar-

barous practice; the more so, as your countrymen,
induced by the man whose bust now stands before you,
have proved that lunatics can be successfully treated
otherwise; and thus you have conferred the greatest
benefit on the unhappiest part of our fellow-creatures.
'The monument which, after my death, I wish to be
erected for me on the Continent, is the practice of non-
restraint; and may this soon be a reality!' These
words I frequently heard from the lips of a man to
whom you so often listened with delight in this same
room, and whose marble effigy we have now to beg you
to accept and place here in perpetual remembrance of
him."

Sir Thomas Watson, in reply, pronounced the following graceful eulogium upon Dr. Conolly :—

" Baron Mundy and Dr. Tuke,—The Fellows of the
College of Physicians, here in full Comitia assembled,
authorise me, their President, to express to you, in their
name and my own, our gratification and gratitude for
the privilege which we owe to your concurrent liberality
of possessing, and of placing permanently within our
walls, the marble bust of one of our body, whose death
we, like you, have but recently been deploring, and
whose memory we, like you, desire to cherish and perpetuate—the late Dr. John Conolly. To you, Baron
Mundy, we offer the tribute of our respect and admiration for your munificence in procuring so costly and
graceful a memorial of your and our departed friend.
And to you, Dr. Tuke, and to the Society represented
by you—the Medico-Psychological Association, to whom

the bust was in the first instance presented by Baron
Mundy,—we have to tender our grateful acknowledgment for the honour you have done this College by
resigning it into our keeping. And again, thanks are
due from us to the Baron for his gracious and ready
consent to that transference. Our sculptured treasures,
gentlemen, are not numerous, but they are tolerably
select. I do not scruple to say that the bust of Conolly
is not unworthy of being associated here with those of
Sydenham, of Mead, of Harvey, and, coming to men of
his own time, of Matthew Baillie, of Halford, of William
Babington. Like theirs, or some of theirs, his name
will go down to a remote posterity, and be reckoned
among those of the greatest and most noble benefactors
to a very suffering portion of the human race, that our
profession and our country have ever produced."

XVIII.

DR. CONOLLY was one of the original members of the *British Medical and Surgical Association,* and with Sir John Forbes, took an active part in assisting their mutual friend Sir Charles Hastings, who originated, and was essentially the *founder,* and, as long as he lived, the animating spirit of the Association.

The Association has proved a great success. It has exercised a powerful influence in promoting the progress of medical science among the members of the profession throughout the whole kingdom. Dr. Stokes, the eminent physician of Dublin, in his address as President of the *thirty-fifth* annual meeting of the Association, held in 1867 (for the first time in Ireland), expresses himself in the following terms regarding its success, and the benefits, social and professional, which have resulted from it:—" Sir Charles Hastings and the far-seeing men who worked with him, kept steadily in view the prospective operation of the Association, not only as a scientific body, but as a means of promoting friendly feelings, by the personal interchange of kindly offices, a means of getting rid of prejudices and of neutralising those corporate jealousies, so long the bane of our profession. Thus they not only hoped, but foresaw that the time would come when the profession would be bound together as a united body, looking ever upwards, and strong in mutual respect and mutual confidence. The experience of the working of the Association warrants us in holding that in a large measure, these anticipations have been fulfilled. We have reason in every respect to be proud of our Institution, proud of it as followers, and therefore as teachers of science, for every man who practises medicine or surgery in a true spirit is himself at once a learner and a teacher. Yet it is not on this ground alone that the British Medical Association is to be considered, for from its very beginning, more than a quarter of a century ago, it has kept other, and, in a sense, higher objects in view. It has in good earnest sought to raise the social status of medicine, by the labours of science on the one hand, and the labours of love on the other. And in this object the records and experience of the past show that it has been successful. It has largely added to the scientific reputation of British medicine and surgery, and it has advanced the social concord of the great body of our brothers who are engaged in the godlike art of healing, which is like mercy, " blessing him that gives, and him that takes."

The success of the Association, in its moral, social, and professional aspects, could not have been expressed in more eloquent terms, nor by a higher authority. Dr. Stokes' views of the influence on the progress and diffusion of medical science effected by the Association

in this country may be found in the character of
the orations at the late remarkable meeting of the
Association in the University of Oxford.   Let any
one compare the orations at the early annual meetings
of the Association, with those delivered at the more
recent meetings, and he will find sufficient evidence
of the immense progress which medical science, in the
largest acceptation of that term, has made throughout
this country since the formation of the Association
upwards of thirty years.

The following extract of a letter to his friend Sir
Charles Hastings shews the interest Dr. Conolly continued to take in the Association long after his health
had greatly failed.   It was written on the eve of the
first meeting of the Association in London :—

" It happened to me, on the 19th day of this month,
to take down the first volume of the *Transactions of
the Provincial Association,* established on the 19th July,
thirty years ago.   Our meeting in the Infirmary on
that day, when I first had the happiness of becoming
acquainted with you,—the memory of those then present,—suggested many, and very varied reflections.
But instead of dwelling on those which are painful
in our mortal state, I consider with pleasure how much
that you anticipated in your opening address, you have
lived to see effected.   Human beings pass away, but the
good they do is immortal, and certainly, my dear and
esteemed friend, you have not lived in vain.   Now that
the thirtieth anniversary is so near at hand, it is impos-

sible not to feel some natural sorrow, when thinking how few of our old provincial members can be present ; and perhaps, some of us may feel a kind of regret that the meeting cannot be exactly of the old provincial kind : —for the memory of past meetings, and all their cordialities, cannot be forgotten. But the more proper feeling to be cherished, is that of satisfaction on seeing the portals of the College of Physicians thrown open to us country doctors, whose first movements attracted little metropolitan consideration. It is most gratifying to me, to think that the *Founder* will be enabled to enjoy this meeting, still vigorous in mind, and still animated by the warm feelings, and cherishing the liberal aspirations, which gave him that influence over men, who were the ornament of our profession, thirty years ago."

Sir Charles Hastings only survived his friend a few months, carrying with him to the grave the esteem and regard of the whole profession, together with that of a large circle of his personal friends.

Dr. Conolly's interest was not confined to medical subjects ; he took a warm interest in everything calculated to promote the advancement of science and literature. He was an active member of the Society for the Diffusion of Useful Knowledge, of which Lord Brougham was president. He contributed numerous small works to the publications of the Society, chiefly on subjects connected with public health and social life. Mr. Charles Knight, the able editor of the publications of the Society, has given the following account of

Dr. Conolly's contributions to the publications of the Society.

" The aid which Dr. Conolly rendered to the diffusion of knowledge was not special or professional. In those departments of what we now call ' social science,' which include the public health in its largest sense, his experience was always working in companionship with his benevolence. In 1831 we were united in the production of a series which was directly addressed to the working classes. Dr. Conolly brought to this useful labour—of which I shall have to make more particular mention—a lucid style, and an accurate conception of the true mode of reaching the uneducated.

" The Useful Knowledge Society had, in November, commenced the issue of a small series entitled, *The Working Man's Companion*, to be published occasionally, at the price of a shilling. The first volume, chiefly prepared by Dr. Conolly, called *Cottage Evenings*, was commended by Dr. Arnold for ' its plain and sensible tone ;' but he is hard upon what he calls its ' cold deism.' He is equally severe upon ' the folly' of a little monthly publication, *The Cottager's Monthly Visitor*, conducted, I believe, by a divine, who was afterwards a bishop."   *   *   *   *

" In the series of the *Working Man's Companion*, we did not neglect the occasion for combating popular errors of a social character, of inculcating the great private duties of cleanliness and temperance as regarded ourselves and our families, and of active benevolence and sympathy for our fellow-creatures.

" Dr. Conolly's little book on cholera was a model of what a popular treatise on the preservation of health ought to be—not leading the delicate and the hypochondriacal to fancy they can prescribe for themselves in real illness ; not undervaluing medicine, but showing how rarely is medicine necessary when the laws of nature are not habitually violated. Of the fatal epidemic that had come amongst us, this wise and kind physician spoke with confidence of its speedy removal, under God's providence, in a condition of society where the principles of cordial brotherhood should more prevail than the miserable suggestions of selfish exclusiveness, where, in fact, the safety of the upper classes depended upon the well-being of the lower." [1]

As an active member of the Committee of this Society, Dr. Conolly was brought into frequent intercourse with Lord Brougham, for whom through life he entertained a great and sincere admiration.

Dr. Conolly was one of the original members of the *Ethnological Society.* He served once as president, and published a paper in the transactions afterwards reprinted in the form of a pamphlet under the title of *The Ethnological Exhibitions of London.* He was also one of the earliest members of the National Association for the promotion of *Social Science ;* and I am informed by my friend Mr. Hastings, the originator of the Association, that Dr. Conolly was for the first two or three years a regular attendant at the monthly meetings of the Council, where he made many useful

[1] *Passages of a Working Man's Life,* vol. ii. pp. 59, &c.

suggestions. He also contributed some valuable papers at the annual meetings of the Association, published in the *Transactions*.

The last association in which Dr. Conolly took an active interest was the *Medico-Psychological Association,* of which he was twice President. When the journal of the Association, the *Asylum Journal,* was established in 1853, he took a warm interest in its success, and although he only contributed to its pages one series of important papers, he never failed to aid the editor with his valuable advice and friendly support. He gave his adherence in a letter to the editor, Dr. Bucknill, of which the following is an extract. (Aug. 31, 1853.) :—

" If I express an interest in the *Asylum Journal,* it will be difficult for you not to think that I am influenced by the very kind things you have been pleased to say of myself. It would be affectation in me to deny that it is most gratifying to me to possess the esteem of honourable men in my own profession, and especially in our own department of it ; and nothing can be more pleasing to me, at my time of life, than to believe, as your kind letter encourages me to do, that after my death, the superintendents of asylums will recollect me as one who sincerely wished to place the insane in better hands than those in which I found them.

" Until I received your letter, I had no distinct idea of what the *Asylum Journal* was to be. Your plan of it seems excellent, and I shall certainly rejoice to see an inde-

pendent journal devoted to psychology, or as Sir Henry
Holland has more plainly and better named our part of
science, mental physiology.

" I should think that analyses of the reports of the
various asylums would be useful in addition to the
subjects you mention: and the mode of government
of different asylums might be usefully examined."

In like manner when the journal, ten years later,
assumed a new name, the *Journal of Mental Science,*
and Dr. C. Lockhart Robertson and Dr. Maudsley
had become editors, Dr. Conolly shows the continued
interest he felt in its success in a letter to Dr. Robertson, of which the following is an extract:—

Jan. 6th, 1863.—" I beg to congratulate you on your
first public appearance as editor of the *Journal of
Mental Science,* No. XLIV. It contains much useful
and valuable matter. Your first paper, on a Middle
Class Asylum for Sussex, will I trust, draw attention to
the great want still existing both there and throughout
England for that class of asylums.

" The Quarterly Report (by Dr. Arlidge) is most
important, and really forms a great step in advance
We have too much wanted the diffusion of useful
knowledge. Our branch of medical science has not
taken its proper place: our great institutions for the
insane are too often governed by persons of moderate
education and narrow views. These things will only
be gradually mended, but never unless mental disorders
become a branch of medical education in our medical
schools."

Dr. Conolly was of opinion that much good might be effected by the public being made acquainted with the condition of our insane and lunatic asylums. "Frequent and liberal discussion," he observed, "of the various subjects connected with lunacy and with asylums, has lately been productive of benefits which will go on increasing, and the varied contents of the *Psychological Journal,* established by Dr. Forbes Winslow, and conducted with great talent and energy, have attracted the attention of many general as well as professional readers to considerations more or less connected with the welfare of the insane." [1]

As the only security for the right treatment of the insane, Dr. Conolly was anxious to see a well educated and able class of superintendents appointed to our asylums and other responsible offices in the department. The following well selected appointments therefore gave him great satisfaction, which he expressed in the following friendly note to Dr. Bucknill, who had asked his advice, when he was a candidate for the office of Lord Chancellor's Visitor of Chancery Lunatics:—

March 21, 1861.—"I am seriously of opinion that your position is such as may make it doubtful whether you should seek any testimonials on applying for the Visitorship. Dr. Hood is also a candidate, and I have had a letter from him expressing himself exactly as you do. Such generous rivalry is gratifying to think of. But I do not consider you so much as rivals as aspirants, whose equal success would gratify us all."

[1] *Treatment of the Insane,* p. 340.

XIX.

IN the early period of his professional life, Dr. Conolly was much engaged in literary works, chiefly medical. The most important of these was the *Cyclopædia of Practical Medicine*, in editing which he was associated with his friends Sir John Forbes and Dr. Tweedie.   He was afterwards associated with the former in originating and editing a still more important work, the *British and Foreign Medical Review*, a journal which had no small influence in improving the state of medical literature in this country.   No critical review was ever conducted on higher principles, and the ability and unflinching honesty with which the medical publications of the time were reviewed, contributed greatly to improve the loose and the often illogical manner in which many of our medical works were written when that review was commenced ; and what was still more important, the principles upon which the study and treatment of disease should be founded, were in that journal ably inculcated : and this and its enlightened articles contributed largely to bring about that more rational and simple method of treating disease, which has happily taken the place of the polypharmic and

so-called active system of treatment which prevailed
generally in this country some forty years ago.

The following account of the influence of the *Review*
on medical science is by a gentleman well qualified to
judge:—

"The effect of this Review on medical literature,
opinion, and practice, has been enormous.   The fair
candid tone of criticism, the careful collection of facts,
the freedom from all party bias, have now been received as the basis of all medical reviewing, and for this
the profession is mainly indebted to Sir John Forbes.
The mere literary merits of the Review were great; its
scientific character was still higher." [1]

The influence of Sir John Forbes's writings in the
Review, and in a small work which he published after
he had ceased to edit the *Review,* entitled *Nature and
Art in the Cure of Disease,* was not limited to this
country.   Dr. Bigelow, one of the most eminent physicians in the United States, writes as follows in a
work which he dedicated to Sir John:—

"I am not willing to leave the subject of Rational
Medicine without more earnestly calling the attention
of the profession in the United States to the admirable
work of Sir John Forbes, already alluded to, on Nature
and Art in the Cure of Disease, of which an American
edition has recently appeared." [2]

---

[1] *Memoir of Sir John Forbes,* by E. A. Parkes, M.D., F.R.S.,
Professor of Military Hygiene in the Army Medical School, &c., &c.

[2] *Exposition of Rational Medicine,* by Jacob Bigelow, M.D.,
Boston, 1858. This allusion to the influence of the writings of Sir
John Forbes will, it is hoped, be excused on the plea of his having

Dr. Conolly's most important published works are those on mental diseases, and on the construction, organization, and management of asylums.   In 1830 he published his *Inquiry concerning the Indications of Insanity,* an able and valuable work, whether we regard the philosophic and judicious plan on which the subject of insanity is viewed, or the ability with which the functions of the healthy mind are examined and analysed as a foundation for the study of its disorders. This part of the work deserves the careful study of all who are engaged or take an interest in the education of youth.   They will find in it the most enlightened advice, conveyed in clear intelligible language, regarding the healthy development of the mind by the well-directed education of its faculties, and the prevention of injury or disease by injudicious, misdirected, or premature exercise of the mind.   To the members of the legal, as well as to those of the medical profession, commencing the study of psychology, this work is well calculated to convey sound views at the outset of their studies; it placed Dr. Conolly in the highest rank as a psychological physician.   He was perhaps the first to point out the rational method of studying disorders of the mind.   Before his time *Insanity* was considered as a *special subject,* apart in its nature from other diseases.   Dr. Conolly showed, however, that deranged states of the mind could only be

been one of the warmest and worthiest friends both of Dr. Conolly and of the author of this Memoir.

properly studied on the same principles which guide us in the investigation of other diseases.

In 1847 he published his work on the *Construction and Organization of Lunatic Asylums.* This work contains full instructions as to the site, arrangement, and government of asylums, and includes much useful information and sound advice on various subjects connected with the health of the insane.

In 1853 he brought out his important work, *The Treatment of the Insane without Mechanical Restraint.* This is a thoroughly practical work, containing the most judicious rules for the application of the non-restraint system, and embraces the whole management of the Hanwell Asylum, during the introduction of the system. It ought to be carefully studied by all who are engaged in the treatment of the insane and the management of asylums, and especially by those who wish to adopt the non-restraint system. Dr. Conolly regarded this as his last work, and expresses the hope that it contains sufficient directions for the guidance of those who desire to adopt the non-restraint system. In referring to its completion he expresses a natural feeling of satisfaction in the following words :—" When the close of active professional exertions is felt to be approaching, and the pressure of that period, ' *aut jam urgentis, aut certe adventantis senectutis,*' becomes perceptible, a natural wish arises in the mind of any man who has been especially engaged in what he regards as a good and useful work, to leave the work, if not finished, yet secure; at least advanced by his labours, and as little incomplete as the shortness of his life and the limitation of his opportunities permit."

Not the least important part of Dr. Conolly's writings are his *Lectures on Insanity*. Among those most deserving notice are two courses delivered in the Royal College of Physicians, London; the *Croonian Lectures;* and a popular course in the Royal Institution.

The apology which Dr. Conolly thought it necessary to make to the College of Physicians, for taking insanity as the subject of his second course of the Croonian Lectures, is worth citing here; it shows how entirely his time and thoughts were occupied in studying the "ruined minds" under his daily observation.

"Having at Hanwell continually before me the spectacle of a crowd of spoiled and ruined minds, my thoughts are so habitually turned to the various phenomena they present, and the various modifications of which they are susceptible, that I should find it difficult to direct them long enough to any other professional subject to justify my addressing you upon it. But the interest which is naturally attached to a malady often mysterious in its origin, most uncertain in its course, and fearful in its results, will doubtless excuse my requesting your attention to it again."

But his most important lectures were those delivered in Hanwell Asylum, and published in the *Lancet*. It is impossible to read these lectures without being impressed with Dr. Conolly's remarkable powers of minute observation, his deep insight into the disordered states of the human mind, and the judicious rules which he laid down for their treatment in the various conditions of health in which they occur. How much more impressive must these lectures have been when the patients, illustrative of them, were under the immediate observation of the student!

In addition to his more formal professional works, Dr. Conolly published many valuable papers in the medical journals, more especially those on *Infantile Insanity*.

A small pamphlet published in 1848, also deserves notice here. It contains most judicious directions as to the plan and organization of a lunatic asylum, founded on the result of his experience and reflection during a residence of nearly ten years in Hanwell Asylum.[1]

A Study of Hamlet, Dr. Conolly's last work, published a few years only before his death, is an elegant philosophical essay on the character of Hamlet, the principal object being to show that Hamlet's was a real, and not a feigned madness, and that such was Shakspeare's intention. Perhaps in none of his works has Dr. Conolly given a greater proof of his powers as a Psychologist than in the minute analysis of Hamlet's mind, to show that his conduct only admits of explanation by his being the subject of actual insanity. Dr. Conolly had long thought over the subject of his essay, return-

---

[1] *A Letter to Benjamin Rotch, Esq., on the Plan and Government of the Additional Lunatic Asylum for Middlesex.*

ing to it in his leisure hours for years, as appears from several letters to his friends. On May 27, 1859, he writes to Dr. Bucknill: " I am extremely obliged by your kindness in sending me a copy of your book, entitled the *Psychology of Shakspeare*. Although I have myself been meditating on Hamlet these eight or nine years past, and once thought of *coming out* this season, I shall not compete with you just now ; and I assure you I read your remarks with great interest. I do not quite, perhaps, take the same view of Hamlet ; but really I feel the study itself so pleasant that I am almost careless of any literary fame connected with authorship. You yourself feel, I observe, how pleasant a thing it is to dwell on the sweet words and wonderful thoughts of Shakspeare.

" I am particularly pleased with your Macbeth, but I shall read the whole work diligently, for I see there is something good in every section. Ophelia is charming, and makes me doubt whether *my* Ophelia is half so fine ; for be it known unto you that *my* book, so resignedly postponed, is *An Examination of the Play and Character of Hamlet.*"

In April, 1860, he writes to his friend Mr. Hunt, of Stratford: " I forget whether I ever told you of my having been engaged, for some years past, in hours not busily employed, in meditating and writing on the *Play and Character of Hamlet*. It has been, as I thought, *finished* over and over again—I mean my essay ; but still I keep fancying I can improve it. Everything that leads me back to Shakspeare and to Stratford is pleasant to me, and I believe I have read every biography of Shakspeare that ever was written."

Certainly no man could have entered on the investigation of the subject who was more fully qualified by his knowledge of the morbid states of the human mind under all their varying phases, and who at the same time combined with his psychological knowledge a more highly cultivated mind, a full acquaintance and appreciation of Shakspeare's works, and a special study of his greatest performance.

" When we revert," says Dr. Conolly, "to his vicissitudes of emotion and passions, and to all the past events of this eventful play, the conviction becomes irresistible, that the madness of Hamlet, therein depicted, has been a real madness. From the first suspicion of the aberration of his mind, we trace the usual results of such an affliction when it occurs in real life." In support of his view he points to a few of the scenes in which Hamlet's conduct is inexplicable on any other view than actual insanity,—his treatment of Ophelia, for instance, in Scene 1, Act II., and more especially in the scene where Hamlet and Laertes meet over her grave : " The picture of madness here is too minutely true, its lights and shades are too close to nature to have been painted as a mere illustration of feigning, and of feigning without intelligible purpose." [1]

" It is impossible," he adds, " to entertain the supposition that Shakspeare would have made so worthless a moral being the principal personage of one of his

[1] *Essay*, p. 265.

noblest compositions, and would have wasted his genius
to adorn such singular moral deformity."

The author of a critical review of Dr. Conolly's
essay,—a great authority,—is of opinion " That the
controversy, whether Hamlet's madness was real or
assumed, may be said to have been brought to a close
by one of the ablest among those in England, who have
had every opportunity of studying the almost innumerable shades through which alienation of the mind
can pass." [1]

The subjoined note, found among Dr. Conolly's
papers, is interesting, because, in addition to the opinion
of an eminent literary man, it contains that of an
actress famous for her delineation of the character of
Ophelia:—

" MY DEAR SIR,—Your book on Hamlet has afforded
me so much pleasure, that I cannot forego the gratification of writing to thank you for it. I have read
probably all that has been written by the best critics
of Germany and France, as well as England, on the
subject, but your treatise seems to me the completest,
and most thoroughly satisfactory exposition of the
character of Hamlet that has ever been attempted.
Based as it is upon a wide experience of mental phenomena, it has infinite practical value, and sets at rest
(to my thinking) the question whether Hamlet's mind
was unhinged or not. My opinion is of no value, but
it may interest you to know that Mrs. Martin (better

[1] *Saturday Review.*

known to the world as Helen Faucit) thinks your demonstration conclusive. Her own study of the play
had long since led her to a similar conclusion—and
when, some years ago, she played Ophelia in Paris, the
question occupied much of her attention. She was
much delighted to find that you corroborate her view
that, Ophelia's madness was in a great measure sym-
pathetic,—induced by that of the man in whom her
whole affections were centred. I have thought this
coincidence of view might be of interest to you to know,
and at all events excuse my troubling you with this
letter. All students of Shakspeare owe you a debt of
gratitude.

                              " THEODORE MARTIN.

" 10th April, 1865."

XX.

BEING desirous of confirming or correcting the opinion
I had formed of Dr. Conolly's position as a writer on
questions of medical psychology, by comparing it with
that of a physician engaged in the branch of the profession to which Dr. Conolly belonged, I applied to my
friend, Dr. Arthur Mitchell, than whom I knew no one
more fully qualified to give a sound opinion on the
subject. This he has kindly done, and has stated his
opinion, and the grounds upon which it rests, so ably
and so clearly, that in place of giving an abstract of his
remarks, I have considered it but justice to him and to
the memory of Dr. Conolly to give them nearly entire.

"The name of Conolly takes rank," Dr. Mitchell
says, "with the names of the foremost men in the
medical profession. It comes up, however, nearly
always, as the name of one who successfully advocated
the humane treatment of the insane ; and it is in this
aspect that the work of Conolly's life is best known.
He is remembered rather as an able and practical
reformer of treatment, than as an analyst of the manifestations of mind. Yet in the best sense of the term
he was a psychologist, and his reputation as a thinker
may well rest on his work on the *Indications of*

Insanity. That work exhibits a sound knowledge of mental operations. It would not, it is true, place its author side by side with some recent writers on medical psychology. It wants the subtlety and fire which their writings display. It deals with the larger and broader divisions of the subject, and avoids that differentiation, which is too apt to become excessive. Minute analysis is of great value and is very desirable; yet the avoiding of it showed sagacity in Conolly, since it was not necessary to the precise aim which he had in view. He goes straight to his object by the shortest and broadest road; and the conclusions he reaches are in unison with those of our best mental philosophers.

" Now and then, throughout the *Indications* there occur passages, which disclose a deep and penetrating knowledge of mind, and which show powers of observation and analysis of a high order. These are *gems,* but it is not to them that the book owes its value : it is the massive *setting* of solid common sense which determines its price.

"So far as language goes, Conolly has written nothing which is not beautiful. In this respect, he has, perhaps, no equal in his own branch of the profession. He commanded a felicitous and elegant way of expressing his thoughts, which will always excite admiration ; and this enviable power he used wisely,—not sacrificing the thought to the turning of the sentence. The consequence is, that in the *Indications* he has produced a book which any man of ordinary education can thoroughly understand. He avowedly uses none

but the simplest terms—those best known and least
open to dispute—and the reader never finds himself
either puzzled or mystified. Few psychological writers
have succeeded in this, and many have lamentably
failed.

" We have in the *Indications,* a book addressed to
the medical profession, but in reality it as much con-
cerns the lawyer and the educationalist. Indeed, no
man will read it and not be the wiser for having done
so, and the better fitted for being the intelligent
guardian of his own mental health. Perhaps the book
deals with the laws regulating the growth and development of healthy mind even more fully than it does
with the signs of invading disease; and the author is
nowhere a wiser psychologist than when he speaks of
the education of the senses, the emotions, the imagination, and the faculties of attention and comparison, and
when he impresses on his reader (which he does over
and over again) that 'the maintaining of a sound state
of mind requires not only attention to its faculties and
to the feelings and emotions, but attention to the
bodily health—a truth too often forgotten in the nur-
ture of children, in the ordering of the studies of youth,
and in the voluntary pursuit of studies or business in
adult age.'

" Whenever Conolly speaks of unhealthy mind, every
'medical man will be sensible of a strength in him from
his having been a physician in general practice, knowing well and by practical observation in what strange
and various ways the manifestations of mind are

influenced by the commoner departures from bodily
health.

"There may not be much in a name, yet I think if
Conolly had called this book by some such title as
' The Mind in Health and Disease,' and if he had
clearly understood himself to be telling *all the world,*
and not simply his professional brethren, how to maintain it in the one state and save it from the other, he
would probably have produced a work which would
have gone through many editions long ere now.

" But although Conolly's reputation as a medical psychologist will rest chiefly on the *Indications,* he is also
most favourably known as an analyst of mind by his
Study of Hamlet, which is a charming piece of philosophical writing—well described as ' full of sense
and scholarship.' I have placed the *Indications* before it, but there are many no doubt who will reverse
the order.

" Dr. Conolly's *Clinical Lectures,* published in the
Lancet in 1845 and 1846, deal chiefly with the external characters of insanity, and I am not aware that
any writer has painted these more truthfully or so
beautifully. In these *Lectures* he makes no attempt
to be profoundly psychological ; he aims rather at
teaching how the different forms of insanity can be
recognised, and being recognised, how they should
be treated ; and in this object he attains an uncom-
mon success.

" The tendency of Dr. Conolly's mind to avoid

differentiation is seen here also, as it was in the *Indications*. His forms of mental disease, indeed, scarcely go beyond mania, melancholia, dementia, and idiocy. Other forms he saw and has described as well as any one, but they presented themselves to his mind not as new or separate forms, but rather as old and familiar ones—modified or complicated. In clinical teaching he seems to have deemed it an advantage to bring as much as possible round one centre, and there are not a few who will acknowledge in this a practical wisdom.

"When he takes the case of a particular patient, and describes the external characters of the disease, and speaks of its history and causes, and tells of the possible and probable issues, and how these may be influenced by treatment,—I scarcely know whether most to admire his broad common sense, or his great knowledge of the subject.

"The same is the case when he refers to the amount of insanity which is but an exaggeration of natural characteristics uncontrolled by a true education, or when he tells how frequently insanity is a disease of debility, and how much this view should regulate its management and treatment. To this last point he often reverts, and there is much sensible writing on the subject in his work on the *Government of Asylums*, when he refers to the influence of diet on recoveries and deaths among the mentally diseased.

"A considerable portion of his published *Clinical Lectures*, however, is devoted to the advocacy of his views on non-restraint. The same is also true of his *Recollections,* published in the *Medical Times and Gazette* for 1862. These *Recollections* are those of a ripe and hale observer ; and the last four relating to juvenile insanity, will increase the usefulness of every medical man who studies them.

" But it was not as a writer on questions of medical psychology that Conolly most influenced public opinion and action. The additions he made to our knowledge of mind, either in a state of health or of disease, are not to be compared in value to his labours as the reformer of treatment. His title to be called a medical psychologist is beyond question ; he observed and studied, and he comprehended the workings of the mind, and knew well the various ways by which it falls into ruin ; and when he wrote on these subjects, he did so in clear and elegant language, which every ordinary man can understand—making his own knowledge easy of access to the many. But if he had never penned a sentence on the stricter topics of medical psychology, the loss to mankind would have been small as compared with what it would have been, had he not written his papers in the *British and Foreign Medico-Chirurgical Review,* his many *Asylum Reports,* his various papers on *Hanwell and Non-Restraint* in the *Lancet* and in the *Medical Times and Gazette,* his Croonian Lectures, his Lectures at the Royal Institution, his book on *Asylum Construction and Government,* and his latest work on the *Treatment of the Insane.*

" I had no personal knowledge of Dr. Conolly. By his writings alone he is known to me, and those of them which I have enumerated appear to reveal the true story of his life's work—that great work which took so much from the misery of a large class of sufferers, and removed at the same time a disgrace from their guardians.

" The treatment of the insane is a chapter in the history of medicine which cannot be read with much pleasure till its closing pages are reached. In these the names of many English physicians stand prominently out, but none so much so as that of Conolly. He was early in the battle-field of reform, and, once there, he never slept but in his armour. By deed, and tongue, and pen, he fought for years a continuous and eager fight. No one can go over the medical literature of the period, and not perceive the truth of this remark. At every step Conolly will be found striking a fresh blow for the cause he had so much at heart. His work on the *Treatment of the Insane without Restraint,* published in 1856, is but the cope-stone to the structure he had long been raising. All that he wrote on the subject was the appeal of an earnest persuasive eloquence, which few men could resist, and which it is his triumph that few men did resist."

It was a great satisfaction to me to find that the opinion which I had previously given of the character and value of Dr. Conolly's works, was as far as it went

endorsed by Dr. Mitchell,[1] whose full and reasoned
opinion will, I feel assured, receive the assent of our
ablest psychological physicians.

In Dr. Mitchell's remark, that if Dr. Conolly had
written his *Indications of Insanity* for the public, the
work would have had a far more extensive circulation and been more generally useful than by its
being intended for the medical profession only, I quite
agree.

In the chapters to which Dr. Mitchell chiefly alludes,
Dr. Conolly shows a power of analysing the operations
of the mind at various periods of life, and as modified
by difference of constitution, which is very remarkable,
when it is remembered that the *Indications* were
written when he was only thirty-four years old.

In addition to what has been said of Dr. Conolly's
writings, it may be useful to notice here, the view he
entertained as to the light in which insanity should be
regarded, and as to the proper method of studying it.
His opinions on Insanity are stated in such clear and
simple language that every well-informed person may
understand them; and the subject is certainly one which
deserves the attentive consideration of every educated
person, in a sufficient degree, at least, to enable him to
perceive the general relations of the sound to the unsound mind, and to know the most frequent causes and
earliest indications of its derangement. Were correct
views more generally entertained of the nature and
causes of mental disease, much of the mystery which is

---

[1] Obituary notice in *Ethnological Transactions*, June, 1866.

attached to it would be cleared away, and as a consequence of this many cases of insanity might be prevented, and many more shortened, by a proper treatment being adopted on the outset of the attack.

After stating that on commencing the study of Mental Diseases, he could obtain little help from the definitions of Insanity, Dr. Conolly proceeds :—" I could not divest myself of the impression that insanity was not understood, only because it was not made the subject of that kind of investigation by which medical men attained a knowledge of any other diseases; and that if they would attend more to the true physiology of the mind, * * * and would also observe the manner in which their own minds were exercised, they would not find it more difficult to mark and to comprehend the departures from the healthy performance of the mental functions, than the deviations from healthy digestion or respiration. What may be said of the difficulty of studying any one of these subjects, may be said of the study of all the rest, and of the mental functions no less than of the corporeal.

" We do not comprehend the nature of the movements or actions on which mental manifestations depend; we do not know how impressions are received and changes effected; but we know the phenomena which result from these movements, from these impressions and changes; we can observe the order, the connection, the effects of the phenomena, and can plainly discern that they are wrought through the agency of corporeal organs. This is the extent of our knowledge of the mental functions, and our knowledge of the bodily functions has precisely the same boundary; we know as much of imagination and memory as we do of respiration and digestion. The limitation of our knowledge does not prevent our observing the functional disorders of the stomach, or of the lungs; nor does any greater obstacle exist in the way of our observation of functional disorders of the brain, however variously produced, which constitutes what we term *mental* disorder. In both cases, we can exercise our senses and our attention on the healthy performance of the function, and on the deviations from healthy performance; and we ought therefore to find no greater difficulty in defining the departure in one case than in the other. The analogy runs through the whole subject.

"It is this application, however, of the ordinary principles of practice, to the cases of mental impairment, which medical men seem to have overlooked. They have sought for, and imagined, a strong and definable boundary between sanity and insanity, which has not only been imaginary and arbitrarily placed, but, by being supposed to separate all who were of unsound mind from the rest of men, has unfortunately been considered a justification of certain measures against the portion condemned, which, in the case of the majority, were unnecessary and afflicting."

Since Dr. Conolly's time, others have followed in their investigations into this subject, the path which he here points out to be the one that must be pursued, if sound conclusions on the nature of insanity are to be reached. He has had many distinguished followers, but no one has suggested a method of studying the physiology and pathology of the mind, which is sounder or better than the one so clearly laid down in this extract from his first work.

CONCLUSION.—In concluding this Memoir of the professional life of Dr. Conolly, I beg to state that it has been my desire to let him describe, in his own clear and elegant words, much of that great work, the accomplishment of which has given him an undying reputation. The large extracts from his works, which this led me to make, disclose that earnestness of purpose and that power in pleading the cause of the lunatic to which his success was so largely due. Few men would have attempted, and fewer could have accomplished, what he did. The suddenness and thoroughness of the first step he took in the introduction of non-restraint, into an asylum containing 800 patients, revealed a man of strong convictions and of courage to act on them. But the completion of his benevolent work was greatly due to other high qualities of mind—self-abnegation, kindliness of heart and manner, and great consideration for those who shared his labours : these did much to secure the steady progress which he made in obtaining followers,—a progress so steady that it was soon true of his own country, that there was scarcely an asylum remaining in it, whose boast it was not that in the treatment of its inmates every form of mechanical restraint had been abandoned. One who knew Dr. Conolly well, writes thus, in describing the aspects of his character just alluded to, as one of the sources of his great success: "Perhaps no one has done so great a work with so little ostentation, so little self-assertion, so much candid appreciation of the merits of others. His public life has been the gain and honour of mankind; and in the noble work which he accomplished he has raised to himself a world-monument, by which men of all lands, through all ages to come, will be taught to remember, not where he died, but where he lived." [1]

A desponding state of mind to which Dr. Conolly was at times subject led him to fear lest the selfish interests of mankind might lead to a reaction, and that much of his work might after all be lost to the world. It seems to have been in some such mood that at the conclusion of his last work he was led to express an anxious hope, that "nothing should be allowed to interfere with its continuation; that no future economy and no delusive theories would ever lead to the abandonment of non-restraint" in the treatment of the insane. "The system," he well adds, "as now established, will form a no unimportant chapter in the history of medicine in relation to disorders of the mind. It has been carried into practical effect in an intellectual and practical age, unostentatiously,

[1] Maudsley, *op. citat.*

gradually, and carefully, and is, I trust, destined to endure as long as science continues to be pursued with a love of truth and a regard for the welfare of man."

In that trust, which forms a fitting conclusion to this imperfect Memoir, every one who has read the history of Dr. Conolly's labours will heartily unite.

————o°o¦°o¦°oo————

APPENDIX.

APPENDIX A.

THE following account of the condition and management of some of the principal asylums on the Continent of Europe has been furnished me by my friend Dr. Arlidge. Much of the information he obtained from personal inspection of those institutions; the rest is derived from various treatises and reports, supplemented by communications kindly forwarded to me in reply to enquiries.

Dr. Arlidge was formerly a pupil of Dr. Conolly at Hanwell, and subsequently, when the resident medical officer of St. Luke's Hospital, succeeded in abolishing the use of mechanical restraint and in ameliorating the condition of the inmates of that institution. Detailed notes on several Continental asylums visited by Dr. Arlidge, appeared in the *Journal of Psychological Medicine*, and he has continued until recently to furnish frequent reports on insanity and asylums in foreign countries to the *Journal of Mental Science*. In 1859 he published a valuable treatise on *The State of Lunacy and the Legal Provision for the Insane, and on Asylum Construction and Organization*: London, John Churchill, New Burlington Street, 1859.

Notes by Dr. Arlidge.

The buildings used for the purpose of public lunatic asylums in the several principal countries of Europe may, in a large proportion, be pronounced ill-suited to their purpose. For the most part they have originally been convents, or monasteries, or fortresses, or private mansions, or otherwise are sections of general hospitals, and have been adapted to their present purpose by various alterations and additions more or less considerable. In Catholic countries converted convents are still largely used as public lunatic asylums. Examples are met with in Florence, Venice (St. Servolo), Sienna, and elsewhere in Italy; in Lyons (Antiquaille), Dôle, Bourg, and other towns of France; in Prague, Leubus, Hildesheim, Siegburg, Brieg, and Aix-la-Chapelle, in Germany. Sonnenstein (Saxony) was originally a fortress, whilst the asylums of Sorau, Lemberg, Stephansfeld, Lyons (St. Jean-de-Dieu), Madrid (Leganez), and Valladolid were private mansions.

Even in England, a century since and less, the prevailing architectural features of convents were adopted by the asylum builders of the time, as appropriate to institutions for the insane; and hence the construction of such hospitals as those of Bethlehem, and St. Luke, and as the rule the introduction of the corridor and cell system in our asylums generally, and, it may be added, in those of other nations. Although a few of the trans-

formed convents may be said to fairly serve the purpose
of asylums, it is doubtless true of by far the greater
proportion, that they are most unfit receptacles for the
insane. This especially holds good of those built within
or immediately outside the walls of towns; in which the
deficiency of space for out-door exercise and employment,
observable in nearly all conventual asylums, more particularly obtains. The additions demanded as necessary
in the transformation of monastic structures to their
novel purpose, have, as a rule, increased their irregularity,
destroyed the original simplicity of design, and curtailed
the previously scanty area for out-door recreation and
work.

Such unfit and more or less miserable establishments
are found at Siegburg, Dôle, Lyons (Antiquaille) Venice,
(St. John and St. Paul female asylum), Sienna and
Hildesheim. The existence of such a building for
lunatics as the Antiquaille, at Lyons,—not only by
reason of its wretched position and construction and its
want of space around it, but also on account of its
immediate connection with the wards for syphilitic
patients and skin diseases—is a disgrace to the second
city of France.

The conversion of private mansions into public
asylums has led to results but little more satisfactory.
The worst specimen probably of such transformation is
the asylum at Sorau, near Frankfort-on-the-Oder, which
is badly arranged, badly situated, and deficient in land;
and yet withal the Prussian Government proposed to
perpetuate this wretched abode for the insane, and to

increase the evil by erecting an additional building in its immediate proximity.

But of the several kinds of accommodation set apart for the insane, that in connection with the buildings and administration of general hospitals is by far the worst. This connection prevails in each of the principal countries of Europe, excepting Sweden and Norway, Denmark and Holland. It is most common in Italy, and Spain, and Belgium, but is also found frequently in Germany and Russia, and more seldom in France. It is seen at Verona, Padua, Rome, Ancona, Trieste, and other Italian cities; at Seville and Saragossa, among many towns in Spain; at Berlin, Breslau, Brünn, Cologne, Danzig, Frankenthal, Gratz, and various other cities of Germany; in three of the hospitals of St. Petersburg, in Moscow, and other Russian towns; at Montpellier, Lyons, and elsewhere in France; in Brussels, and most other towns of Belgium. Of such asylums or lunatic wards, those at Verona, Padua, Ancona, Saragossa, and Berlin are among the worst.

Turning to foreign asylums specially constructed as such, an immense diversity in the fitness of their sites, construction, and internal arrangements exists. The oldest of them date from the close of the last century, and betray in their structure the opinions prevailing in the several countries at the time of their construction, respecting the wants of the insane and their safe keeping. Alessandria, in Piedmont, possesses an asylum erected in 1785, but condemned by its present medical director as quite unfit for its purpose; and Spain, which has altogether lingered so far behind in the march of improvement, boasts of a noble asylum, palatial, architecturally viewed, built at Toledo in 1793, but unsuited to its purpose by its town site and its general prison-like arrangements internally. Turin is an instance of a specially designed asylum, projected on a considerable and somewhat expensive scale some sixty years ago, but now rightly regarded as a totally unfit residence for lunatics.

Among asylums which have been erected within the last thirty years, and may be quoted as the best,—*i. e.*, those of which we can express an opinion from personal observation or from descriptions and drawings—are Auxerre, Marseilles, Quatre Mare (Rouen), and Grenoble, in France ; Ghent, in Belgium ; Meerenberg, in Holland ; Illenau, in Baden ; Halle, in Saxon Prussia ; Sachsenberg, in Mecklenberg-Schwerin ; Chambéry, in Savoy ; Heppenheim, in Hesse ; and Aarhuus, in Jutland. To this list many newly constructed asylums ought doubtless to be added.

Omitting the two great hospices of Paris, the Salpêtrière, with 1431 female, and the Bicêtre with 980 male lunatics, the largest asylum known to us is that at Maréville, near Nancy, which contains 1200 inmates. The new Vienna asylum affords room for 800, and the wretched Antiquaille at Lyons for 700, the like number being also found at Lemberg. Marseilles provides for 600, and as many are found in the crowded wards of Stephansfeld, near Strasburg. These are examples of Continental asylums of unusual magnitude, and the concurrent opinion of foreign psychiatrists is that they are too large, whether viewed with reference to the well-being of their inmates or to economical considerations. The maximum number desirable and advantageous is generally fixed at 500; and the prevailing practice is to build for a smaller number.

It would be fortunate for this country and its insane population, could the visiting magistrates of asylums be induced to listen to the concurrent opinions of medical men who are charged with the treatment of the insane, and to learn that the rational object of collecting insane people together is not safe custody, proper feeding and clothing, but cure. In England, unhappily, this lesson is unheeded, and the current principle of action is, simply to put lunatics in asylums (hence properly enough named), in order that they may be kept from doing harm and be out of harm's way. It is not surprising, therefore, that lunatics are ever accumulating, and that wing after wing, or storey upon storey, is added to the already overgrown establishment. Some day, it is to be hoped, the public will awaken to the conception that hospitals are needed for the treatment of insanity, that such hospitals must not be expanded into receptacles for incurables, and, lastly, that they must have a sufficient and efficient medical staff.

In noting the population of the public asylums of the Continent generally, it should be borne in mind that, unlike most those of England, they are of a mixed character, affording accommodation to one or two classes of pensioners, *i. e.*, private persons able to pay for their maintenance more or less liberally, and such as find their

way into the private asylums of this country—besides the
indigent or pauper classes.   These pensioners are furnished with superior accommodation, in a more or less
separate wing or section of the institution, under special
organization and management.   In some measure,
therefore, the department of the pensioners is a distinct
establishment, and the proportion of its inmates might
fairly be deducted from the general total of the asylum
inhabitants when comparing the population with that of
an English public institution.

There is, moreover, a great contrast between English
and foreign asylums in the extent of medical supervision
thought necessary.   In England the efficiency of medical
superintendence appears to be regarded as highly elastic
and capable of immense extension.   Or rather, it may
be more correctly stated that the value of the medical
man, *quoad* his medical character, is estimated at a very
low rate.   In short, the medical superintendent of most
English asylums is simply an overseer or overlooker, and
his place might be filled by a layman of moderate intelligence, did not the law require medical qualifications, and
did not accidents and emergencies arise in such establishments for which medical skill is called in requisition.

But, on the Continent, the opposite principle obtains.
The necessity of a medical staff somewhat in proportion
to the number of inmates is recognized, and the value of
medical observation and of individual treatment and
supervision are duly appreciated.   Even in small asylums
of from one to two hundred inmates, the physician-in-
chief has at least one if not two assistants, and in many

instances, moreover, a pharmacien is added to the staff.
In numerous institutions, moreover, the medical element
is further strengthened by the presence of one or more
" internes," and the value of asylums as training schools
for the medical profession thereby utilized.

In a very few foreign institutions for the insane,
found almost exclusively among those that are merely
sections of general hospitals, but also including a few
others in the hands of religious communities, *e. g.*, the
asylums of Caen and Bourg, no medical superintendent
is resident, and the constant supervision of the patients
is committed to an inferior non-medical officer, to an
" interne," or to the members of the brotherhood or
sisterhood, as the case may be.   It is not to be wondered
at, therefore, that in such establishments the condition
of the patients is most neglected and most wretched.
The hospital sections for lunatics at Verona, Padua,
Brescia, and Venice, and the asylum belonging to the
sisterhood at Caen may be quoted in illustration.   The
last-named institution is a singular instance of toleration
in France—a circumstance attributable to the unwillingness of the Government to interfere with privileges
accorded in a previous generation to a religious sisterhood, although those privileges are incompatible with
the welfare and happiness of those entrusted to their
charge, because it is a religious community, and because
interference might offend the Church and the religious
feelings and prejudices of the votaries of the Church.
Did the French Government feel itself free to act, the
toleration of such a receptacle for the insane would at

once be revoked; for it is universally condemned by the psychiatrists of France. Its patients are simply farmed out to the nuns, who assume all authority in the organization and management of the inmates, exercise severe restraint, seclusion, and penance at their discretion; oppose improvements as antagonistic to their cherished creed and prejudices; and, by way of apology, to supply medical treatment, engage the services of two physicians in general practice, resident in the town, at a distance from the institution, to visit daily, to prescribe for the sick. It may be gathered from these remarks that the building is unfit structurally for an asylum; that restraint is much practised, and recreation and employment very limited. Moreover, the nuns are schoolmistresses, and on the same premises have a large boarding-school for girls.

The manner in which the duties of the resident physician is performed in foreign asylums is, with respect to medical and dietetic details, usually very thorough. The several wards are gone through and their individual occupants spoken to, encouraged, put to work, or tempted to amusement, and, when needed, prescribed for medically; the assistants or internes noting down the orders for medicine, diet, and other particulars, from the lips of the physician whom they follow in his rounds. His professional position and duties are not lost sight of, or overwhelmed by those of the general steward and overseer; whilst his medical supervision and the carrying out of treatment, derive completeness and efficiency from the aid furnished him in the person of qualified assistants.

One visit daily to all the patients is the universal custom, but a second, of a more general character, or devoted more especially to particular cases under observation, is almost always made. At other hours one or other assistant is called upon to make supplementary visits, and to superintend and carry out the directions of his superior in the wards and grounds.

By this complete medical organization, opportunity is given for securing that individual observation and treatment of the insane, which every writer on insanity insists upon as necessary to asylum usefulness and to curative treatment. It contrasts strongly with that commonly found in English asylums, where, owing to the deficient medical staff, the position and importance of the ordinary attendants acquire an undue preponderance; where these servants are the eyes and hands of the superintendent in medical as well as in other matters more cognate to their position and knowledge.

In a few instances, for the most part occurring in France, the general management of the asylum is lodged in the hands of a director, who, as a rule, is not a medical man. In such institutions consequently, the physician is a subordinate officer in all matters save those purely medical. This position of the physicians, and the consequent divided authority in asylums, is most justly condemned by all the leading psychiatrists of the Continent, and it is hoped that the arrangement will be, ere long, given up wherever now found. Although such divided status and authority must be condemned, an error in the opposite direction is made in English

asylums, by overburdening the medical superintendents
with details of house and farm management, whereby
their medical character becomes more or less merged
in, and sacrificed to, the duties of house and farm-
steward.

The greater completeness of the medical organization
of foreign asylums being admitted, the question arises
wherein does its value appear? The first and most
important success that an asylum can show,—*i. e.*, if an
asylum is to be regarded as a place for the cure as well
as for the detention and security of lunatics—is the
number of cures effected within it. Into this question,
however, we cannot here enter: suffice it to say that
foreign asylum physicians draw up statistical tables
with much diligence and pride, to prove that they are
more successful in the treatment of their insane than
are our English superintendents. But, be this as it may,
it is worth while to point out some of the obstacles to
success that encompass foreign psychiatrists, and from
which our own asylum physicians are more or less
exempt. These obstacles are found in the structures
used for asylums, in the state of the law and finances,
and in the intelligence and feeling of the country,
and lastly in the existence of professional and popular
prejudices. The first of these calls for most notice.

Esquirol very rightly and forcibly called an asylum
an instrument of cure. Regarded as such, its efficiency
will depend very largely on its degree of perfection in
structural arrangements and internal appliances for the
special wants of the insane. The previous remarks on

foreign asylums indicate how large a majority of these institutions are in these respects ill-adapted for their purpose.

That a greater advance has not taken place in the architectural and structural arrangements as well as in the details of management, in foreign asylums, must be in a considerable measure attributed to the inertness, prejudice, ignorance, and obstinacy of governing bodies, and not to the want of enlightened and humane views on the part of the physicians.   In France the system of centralization and the appointment of asylum inspectors has done much, under the influence of the law requiring every Department to provide asylum accommodation for its own lunatics, to improve the character of its institutions for the insane.   In Germany, the paternal action of many of the principalities has secured satisfactory provision for a considerable proportion of its lunatic population ; but, curiously enough, the country in Germany which prides itself most on its intellectual and political superiority, Prussia, is the most negligent of the claims of its insane, and presents in most of its principal institutions for them the grossest defects and unfitness.   The Berlin " Charité " Lunatic Hospital for curables, the Arbeithaus, also in Berlin, for incurables, are, especially the latter, among the worst abodes destined for lunatics on the continent of Europe, and a disgrace to Prussia.   Breslau has only a small section of its general hospital for recent cases ; and Leubus, intended rather for private than for pauper patients, is a converted monastery indifferently arranged and fitted for its object, and situate in a swampy country. The Sorau Asylum is a most sorry specimen, an altered and ill-suited private house, with very restricted gardens, badly situated close to the town, in an undesirable valley. Nor will the additional buildings supply the necessary and suitable accommodation. Eastern Prussia and Pomerania, and the Rhenish provinces have no satisfactory asylum buildings, and the only laudable attempts in the powerful Prussian monarchy, to erect establishments in harmony with the progress of psychiatrical knowledge, are found at Halle, in Saxon Prussia, and Langerich in Westphalia. On the contrary, in Austria, very rapid improvement has gone on, and many new and commendably arranged asylums erected, as at Brünn, Ybbs, Hermannstadt, and Vienna; whilst several others have been in a great measure rebuilt, as those at Gratz and Linz.

In Italy the political state of the country has greatly hindered the course of asylum improvement. A new asylum is building or built on the island St. Clemente, to accommodate the insane females heretofore imprisoned in the wretched hospice of St. John and St. Paul, in the middle of the city of Venice. But unhappily some misunderstanding or ill-feeling subsists between the local authorities in several provinces and the medical officers of asylums, so that the latter are held in little esteem, and are thwarted in their plans by councils from which they are intentionally excluded. Such are the statements conveyed to us by the physicians themselves in their published works and periodicals.

The Scandinavian nations and the Dutch have followed closest in the wake of England in the endeavour
to improve the condition of the insane. The asylum of
Meerenberg, in Holland, has acquired much fame from
its structural arrangements and excellent management,
and the Danish institutions possess considerable merit.
Of the latter, the one near Aarhuus, in Jutland, is an
excellent example; the other two, one in Zeeland and
the other in Fünen, are likewise of recent construction
and well spoken of. In Sweden and Norway the provision for the insane has, within a few years, been entirely reorganized, and new provincial asylums erected,
honourable to the kingdom.

In Russia, thirty years ago, the need of improved
dwellings for the insane was fully recognised, and was,
in some places, as, for example, in St. Petersburg, met
by the erection of costly buildings after the best models
then known. The asylum of the Russian capital accommodates 500 patients; but besides this special institution, further accommodation for the insane is given in
sections of three of the general hospitals; an arrangement, it is needless to say, unsatisfactory in the highest
degree, and one which should no longer continue. At
Moscow is a special asylum for 200, and at Kasan,
Dorpat, and Vilno, new asylums are constructed. In
Finland the public provision for the insane is both
deficient and bad.

Belgium has been very slow in carrying out the
reform of its lunatic institutions. The state of Belgian
lunatics, and of the places in which they are detained,

has been painted in very dark colours by the Commissioners appointed to inquire into those matters; and the renowned asylum physician of the country, M. Guislain, very shortly before his death reflected strongly upon the tardy and imperfect measures proposed or carried out to ameliorate the condition of the insane.

In Switzerland some well-directed attempts have been made to remedy the neglect of past years, and new asylums have been erected in several of the cantons. A modern one at Berne is well spoken of; but at Geneva is an old building not in keeping with the accepted principles of asylum construction and arrangement, and which should at once be replaced by a suitable establishment.

But besides structural details, the site and surroundings of very many Continental asylums are also most unfit. A large proportion are situated in cities, abutting upon streets, and many are in too close proximity to towns and public roads. Such sites imply deficient courts and gardens, restricted space for workshops and the absence of agricultural employment; a list of deficiences, however, existing not only in such town-placed asylums, but even in some situated in the open country.

Of asylums of considerable magnitude situate within or in the outskirts of towns, may be enumerated for example, those of Rome, Florence, Bologna, Venice, Geneva, Turin, Montpellier, Dôle, Lyons, Prague, Hildesheim, Berlin, Sorau, Toledo, &c. Of these, however, some are very much better off for space,—for exercising courts and gardens. At Rome, where reform in matters

R

generally is heresy, the energy of the chief physician
of the lunatic section of the great hospital of S. Spirito,
which in past years was one to point at as exhibiting
the worst defects of an asylum, has triumphed in
achieving great ameliorations, particularly by the addition of courts and gardens for exercise and out-door
employment. Among the other asylums enumerated,
those at Florence, Venice (the female asylum), Turin,
Bologna, Berlin, Lyons, and Toledo, may be instanced
as most wanting in space for the use of their unfortunate inmates; a deficiency which, when rightly appreciated and considered in conjunction with their
architectural faults, should compel their abandonment
as unfit places for treating lunatics.

Again, the utility of foreign asylums considered as
instruments of treatment is lessened by professional
and popular prejudices, by the ignorance and perverse-
ness of public authorities, and by meagre grants for
their maintenance. Popular prejudice also shows itself
abroad more than in England in reference to the fear
entertained of lunatics, to the notion that they need be
securely guarded and are untrustworthy. Hence the
great frequency of walled exercising courts, which in
some cases are mere bare yards, the protection of
windows by iron bars, the very common denial of
knives at meals, and the distrust often shown in with-
holding tools employed in various trades. The walled
courts necessarily shut out views and have at best a
prison-yard character, and it strikes the English visitor
as curious that the formation of sunk fences has not

been in numerous instances where quite available, resorted to.

To prejudice, both professional and public, must be
attributed the denial to the patients of many conveniences and comforts found generally in English
asylums, calculated to exercise a calmative influence,
to awaken agreeable impressions, and to foster self-
control and self-respect. Thus in many foreign asylums
we meet with bare, unadorned walls in corridors and
day-rooms; the absence of comfortable seats, and of
arrangements for personal cleanliness; the scanty supply
or well-nigh deprivation of books, papers, and games;
the prevalent misgiving of bringing the two sexes
together on occasions of general recreation; the limited
permission to attend religious worship; and, in general,
the more restricted and prison-house-like routine, and
the display of strength and security in the fittings
and arrangements at large.

Still, great variety obtains in different Continental
asylums in respect to these particulars. Some institutions, as for example that at Auxerre, in their *tout
ensemble*, rival in internal conveniences and comforts
English asylums. Others, such as Brescia, Lyons,
Venice, and Berlin, differ *toto cœlo*. Moreover, different
institutions affect different amusements and occupations
for their inmates. At Sonnenstein, gymnastics are
much cultivated; in a few, theatricals are patronized;
in a larger number, dances and musical meetings; whilst
billiards, cards, and dominoes are played in the majority of the better class of foreign establishments. It

should be noted, however, that the too common practice is to furnish means of amusement and recreation to the pensioners or paying patients only or chiefly; the indigent being left pretty much to devise amusements for themselves, and in consequence often to bring down upon themselves the indignation of their doctors and attendants for the indiscreet kind resorted to.

Employment of some sort or other, dictated somewhat as to kind by that most pursued in the district served, and by the surroundings and resources of the institution, is encouraged in all but a few of the very worst foreign asylums. Weaving is carried on at Lyons and Aversa; but the staple employment in such establishments generally, where practicable by the possession of ground, is garden and field labour. In a few instances, indeed, particularly at some of the French asylums, among which those of Auxerre and Maréville might be instanced by some critics, the labour of the patients has been pushed to an extreme; the ambition of the directors being to reduce to a minimum the subvention required from the communes and departments, by means of the profit derivable from the work of the inmates.

There is always greater facility of supplying occupation to females, and this explains the general superiority noticeable in the sections of asylums occupied by them. And it would not be right to pass unnoticed the very excellent work-rooms for women, and the admirably kept and arranged store-rooms for clothes and linen, as met with in the great majority of Continental asylums, and which constitute, indeed, in some instances, the only redeeming feature in the otherwise miserable establishment.

Even in institutions where no systematic or organized labour is in operation on account of the absence of means in the shape of workshops and of ground for cultivation, the physicians are very sensible of the sad disadvantage thereby entailed. Of late years in several cases the strong representations made to the authorities by them have secured the possession of land at a greater or less distance from the asylum, which the patients are daily sent to cultivate, and where, likewise, in several instances, a certain number have been located in a supplementary building, " annexe," or " succursale." Examples occur at Leyme, Pau, Dôle, and elsewhere in France.

The preceding sketch of the state of foreign asylums will prepare the reader to expect that, when viewed from an English stand-point, the treatment pursued, particularly in relation to the deprivation of the liberty of patients by seclusion and mechanical fastenings, is far from being what it should be.

Seclusion is often talked about abroad as pre-eminently the English fashion of subduing excitement without having recourse to mechanical coercion. But, as a result of personal observation, seclusion, or the shutting up of patients, mostly singly, but sometimes several together, prevails to a much larger extent in foreign than in English asylums. A group of refractory patients may be seen, particularly in the smaller

miserable asylums of Italy, shut in a room by themselves, but privileged it may be to rave and shout at
the barred window or the open-barred door. And
when solitary confinement is enforced, it is more frequently than not accompanied by mechanical restraint
of the patient. It may be also put as a general statement that seclusion is not so entirely placed under the
control of the medical officers, nor are its frequency
and duration registered, as in this country. The
proportion of cells in many Continental asylums is
considerable, especially in those erected on the model
of our old asylums ; nevertheless, as a rule, dormitories
are of more frequent occurrence, and relatively of
larger dimensions than in England. Examples of very
large dormitories occur in the Hospice of St. Jean-de-
Dieu, near Lyons, and in the Florence Asylum, the
dormitories containing severally 50 to 70 beds.

M. Renaudin, formerly director of Maréville, and
more recently of Dijon Asylum, denounces cells altogether, and has entirely abolished them where he has
had the power, as at Maréville. But he has made few
converts to his extreme views, for there is a general
concurrence among foreign physicians that a certain
proportion of single rooms is desirable in an establishment for the insane, and in this point they are in
harmony with our own countrymen.

Until the last few years the so-called " English system " of non-restraint had not an acknowledged disciple
on the continent of Europe. It was scouted as an
absurdity and a trick or deception. But a handful of

wiser men determined to examine for themselves what non-restraint really is, and how it is carried out in the British Islands; and having seen and satisfied themselves of its reality, its nature and practicability, have become advocates of the system in their several native lands. Morel of Rouen, Griesinger of Berlin, whose death medical science has to deplore, Meyer of Göttingen, Dr. Augusto Tebaldi of Italy, and Dr. Salomon of Malmö, Sweden, and last, not least, Baron Mundy, are the leaders in this band. Dr. F. Fusier, of the Chambéry (Savoy) Asylum, may likewise be reckoned a convert, for according to the testimony of Dr. Carmichael, who visited the Savoy institution in 1863, "no camisoles are used, nor was any form of restraint to be seen."—(*Journal of Mental Science*, April, 1864, p. 5.) At Malmö Asylum, restraint has been given up for four years, and it was also in 1864 that Morel entered the lists as an advocate of non-restraint, and has used his best energies to put the plan into execution at Rouen, though beset with difficulties from structural unfitness and defective control over the entire organization of the institution.

The extent of coercion in the different asylums of Europe varies very considerably. In the most wretched hospital lunatic wards, of Italy pre-eminently, restraint in all forms is the rule. Continuous confinement in bed by the aid of belts, straps, wide bandages across the body, and by fastenings for hands and feet to the bedstead, is there to be witnessed. For others, confinement in ingeniously-made chairs whereby all movement nearly, save of the head, is abolished; for a more favoured number, camisoles, belts, handcuffs, hobbles, and leathern muffs or thick gloves restraining all movements of the hands and fingers. Happily such severe restraint is very rare out of Italy and Spain; but if M. Berthier is correct in his notes on French asylums, a far too near approach to such barbarous treatment may still be found in the Caen Asylum under the immediate care and management of a holy Sisterhood, jealous of intruders within their asylum, as well as of doctors; for as with such religious Roman communities in general, so with them, insanity is a spiritual disease, in which the enemy of mankind is greatly concerned, and consequently it is but charity to restrain the evil spirit, even at the cost of suffering to the body.

A sad amount of restraint was however to be seen in other French, and likewise in not a few German asylums. At Lyons, Montpellier, Bourg, and Stephansfeld, confinement in bed and in chairs, restraint belts, camisoles night and day; and the like measures were resorted to in many German asylums, in Berlin, Prague, Leubus, Illenau, Hildesheim, Siegburg, and elsewhere. In Berlin, under Ideler, the restraint used at La Charité was very severe and prolonged. But in other institutions again, mechanical restraint was reduced to a minimum; among such may be adduced the asylums of Auxerre, Quatre-Mare (near Rouen), Dôle, and Maréville, in France; Aarhuus (Jutland), Meerenberg (Holland), St. Servolo (at Venice), Perugia, &c.

Excepting Sweden, Denmark and Holland, France
has advanced more than any other country on the
Continent in the amelioration of the condition of
the insane. In that country the rigour of treatment
has been much softened; greater liberty allowed to the
patients in asylums, more pains taken to occupy and
divert the mind. In Germany a rigid drilling and
discipline, a painfully visible order, is perceptible,
placing each individual mind in bonds, and suppress-
ing its natural lightness and elasticity. Repression
appears to be the order of the day, and it would seem
that the aim is to conform and transform each mind
under treatment to a given standard or model, the
development of pure psychological reflection in the
brain of a metaphysician. It is in Germany more than
in France that non-restraint is misunderstood and
abused as a cheat.

The old prevailing dread of the insane, and an
anxiety to obviate evils, possibly existant only in the
imagination of physician and attendants, are so strongly
rooted in the minds of many asylum superintendents,
that if their courage holds out by day in taking off
instrumental restraint, it fails them at night, especially
in the case of newly-admitted patients, who are as a
matter of routine made secure as imagined, when in
bed, by some mechanical contrivance.

In Holland, Dr. Conolly's teachings have been most
cordially accepted; the legal protection and public
provision for the insane have been secured by enlightened laws, and new buildings erected throughout

the country for its lunatic population. From accounts received, restraint is little resorted to, and in some asylums, laid aside altogether. As already noticed, at Malmö, in Sweden, non-restraint is fully adopted as the principle ; in Norway, as at the Christiania City Asylum, Dr. Wing, the physician, is unfortunately impressed with the belief that mechanical coercion is not only necessary to restrain violence, but also useful as a means of correction ; in Denmark, as Dr. Selmer of the Jutland Asylum reports, the constant desire is to reduce restraint as much as possible. At the same time he is of opinion that " there are cases incompatible with the humane spirit of the non-restraint system carried out to the very letter."—(Extract from a letter, May, 1867).

A minor point that may be referred to is the long detention in bed, common in Continental asylums. At five or six o'clock in the evening the patients are got to their bedrooms, and there kept until about six o'clock in the morning. This circumstance in a measure explains the abundance of cases of dirty habits, and the need of the greater resort to mechanical restraint by night than by day.

Paris Asylums.—In the course of the preceding remarks on foreign asylums, no special reference has been made to the great public establishments for the insane in Paris,—the Salpêtrière and Bicêtre,—so well known to physicians by the labours of Pinel, Esquirol, Ferrus, Falret, Baillarger, and others, inasmuch as they may now be reckoned among institutions of the past.

Their irregular structure, deficient appliances in the
way of space for recreation and of means for promoting
occupation, their association with contiguous charitable
foundations, and other and many defects as receptacles
for the insane, are facts that have been pointed out for
a long series of years by many writers. At length a
resolution was taken to abolish them, except as asylums
for old people, demented, and others, and to provide
for the insane of the Department of the Seine in several
new asylums, situated within a convenient distance
from Paris. This step was further called for by the
constantly augmenting number of lunatics. At the
present time a central institution in Paris, and three
new asylums, containing each 600 patients, are established. The " Bureau Central " constitutes the centre
of organization and general control. It serves for the
primary reception of patients, for the close observation
and examination of their cases by the two physicians
attached to it, prior to deciding on the particular
asylum to which they shall be sent. It also contains
the general offices connected with the government and
management of the several departmental asylums.
Patients are not detained there except perhaps for a
few days; unless indeed, some medico-legal question
has to be decided with reference to them.

Of the outlying asylums, that of St. Anne was the
first constructed and opened (May, 1867), on the site
of the old farm of St. Anne, which served, under the
auspices of Falret, as an annexe of the Bicêtre many
years. This asylum is set apart for the treatment of

recent cases. The other two new institutions are destined for convalescents, for chronic and for some sub-acute cases of insanity. They are provided with more land than St. Anne's for the employment and recreation of their inmates, with workshops, detached buildings for special cases, and with châlets, distributed here and there on the estates, calculated to rally their occupants to the conditions of ordinary life.

To each of these new establishments is also attached a department for private cases, drawn from the middle class of society, and charged with the cost of their maintenance and treatment.

At present, infirm and very chronic cases, together with epileptics and idiots, will be detained at the Salpêtrière and the Bicêtre. It is, however, the intention to hereafter erect special asylums both for epileptics and for idiots.

The acreage of St. Anne's Asylum is only 35 acres; but the new asylum, Ville Evrard, near Neuilly-sur-Marne, possesses 750 acres, and that of Vaucluse, 300 acres. Each institution, as before noted, is intended to accommodate 600 inmates, 300 of each sex. The "Bureau Central" has 44 beds,—22 for each sex. It is under the immediate supervision of the Inspector-General of the Department and of two physicians. It is proposed to organize within it a department for giving gratuitous advice in mental disorders.

The medical staff at St. Anne's consists of two physicians, two internes specially engaged, and two others subordinate, a surgeon, and a pharmacien. At Ville

Evrard and Vaucluse the staff is composed at present of a medical director, two internes and a pharmacien; but the project is entertained of adding a physician-adjoint to it.

The only form of mechanical restraint employed in these new establishments is the camisole. This, moreover, is resorted to only in exceptional cases, and every effort is made to abolish this last remnant of coercion.

Gheel.—In a sketch of Continental asylums, a brief notice is due to the insane colony of Gheel,—a development of the middle ages which, of late years, has exercised an immense influence everywhere upon the treatment of the insane. Its system cannot be quoted as exemplifying the advantages of non-restraint; for restraint prevailed there largely, and is still too much in vogue; but it has served as a standing argument against the only principle which has taken hold of the public mind with regard to dealing with the insane; that, viz., of shutting them up in asylums. It has been the means of illustrating to what extent the insane may be mixed up with the sane, and be permitted to enjoy the common amenities of life; of demonstrating the wide scope that may be given to the employment of lunatics, particularly in out-door labour. It has fostered the development of the "cottage system" in connection with "close asylums;" has furnished the example, so successfully copied in Scotland, of boarding chronic cases in cottage dwellings, under due supervision; and has encouraged the establishment of medico-agricultural institutions for the insane, wherein its leading features are copied. And it has yet much to accomplish :—much in its own internal organization, and still more in further modifying the long-cherished notions and prejudices respecting the requirements of lunatics that have grown up under the shadow of the old system of aggregation and seclusion, of gigantic asylums and armies of keepers—a system confessedly defective and unequal to the demands of the insane.

The preceding remarks on Continental asylums repose on personal observation in respect to a very large number of those institutions. They were visited in 1855, and a few of them at later periods. It may be objected that great improvements have been carried out in the lapse of thirteen years. Of this happily there can be no question ; yet the portraiture attempted reflects in the main the actual state of things in the several countries and asylums enumerated, the writer having taken pains to inform himself, as far as practicable, by reference to periodical literature and to modern publications, with the changes that have taken place in them, and to give credit for the improved state of things.

In conclusion, it may be remarked, that the hindrance to the advancement of the more humane views of treatment, as advocated by Dr. Conolly, among the several nations of the Continent, is chiefly attributable to the tardiness with which foreign asylum physicians make use of the opportunities afforded them of visiting our

asylums, and of making themselves practically conversant with what non-restraint, as carried out in them,
actually is.   Instead of following the example of Morel
and others, in entering our asylums and watching in
their wards by day and night the details of daily life
and management in operation, they too largely content
themselves with setting up an ideal of non-restraint,
fashioned after their own imaginations, and then
valiantly demolish it to their own satisfaction.   They
sometimes seem to consider that the casting away all
instruments of mechanical coercion is the sum and
substance of English non-restraint, and so mistake
the part for the whole.   They have to learn that non-
restraint implies, besides this one feature, a multitude
of details.   It implies an appropriate building on a
suitable site, ample surrounding space for gardens and
fields, and shops for employment and recreation ; internal arrangements calculated to solace and divert the
mind diseased and to occupy it in some useful direction,
as well as to provide for all the decencies and comforts
of life ; the presence of well-paid attendants, entirely
under the control of the medical superintendent, and
animated by a like spirit with him of self-denial, self-
devotion and kindness, and last, and above all, a superintending physician, unfettered by others in the medical,
hygienic, and moral management of the institution, in
possession of a calm yet vigorous and determined mind,
thoroughly imbued with the conviction that his patients
are best treated by humane means without coercion,
and who, in fine, is penetrated, so to speak, by a love
of the insane.

APPENDIX B.

FOR the following sketch of our colonies, in relation to their treatment of the insane, I am indebted also to Dr. Arlidge, who collected the greater part of the information and arranged it in its present form. My best thanks are due to the officers of the Colonial Office, who supplied me readily with all the information on the subject which they possessed. It will be seen that in the greater number of our colonies there is much room for improvement in the character of the asylums and general treatment of the insane. The West Indies is in the most deplorable state of all; and the spirit of improvement exhibited by our other colonies, seems to have no existence there. The sketch is very imperfect, but will form the basis I hope of a much more satisfactory report a few years hence.

BRIEF NOTES ON THE BRITISH COLONIAL ASYLUMS.

With few and recent exceptions, the asylums existing in the several colonies belonging to this country are unsatisfactory and unfit receptacles for the insane. Their general history may be thus represented. Cases

of insanity in the early career of the colony have been
transferred for security sake to gaols and to hospitals
without any special arrangements to meet their requirements. Soon the accumulation of such cases, and the
inconveniences caused thereby, have dictated the necessity of their separation from other inmates, and, for this
purpose, some particular division of the gaol, and a
distinct ward or collection of wards in the hospital, has
been set apart for their accommodation. This connection of lunatic wards with general hospitals, with
convict establishments and with gaols, has been kept
up in several colonies to the present day, and, it need
not be said, is bound up with well-nigh all those conditions that are inimical to the well-being of the insane.
In a considerable number of the colonies the insane
have been collected in particular buildings, but in very
few instances have such buildings been especially constructed for the purpose they are devoted to; nor has
the condition of their inmates in many of them been
much better than that of those lodged in the wards of
hospitals and gaols.

A circular despatch, emanating from the Colonial
Office and addressed to the Governors of Colonies,
called forth a brief Report, in 1863, on the several
colonial hospitals and lunatic asylums then in existence,
based upon returns made by their officials. A more
melancholy and painful account than this presented
could scarcely be imagined. It reflects disgrace as
well on the parent country as on the colonies. The
colonial hospitals are, with few exceptions, reported as

S

bad, but the asylums as worse. "They suggest the impression that they are regarded too much as a means of relief from a troublesome class, without care for curative treatment." The sites are very frequently objectionable: the buildings often old barracks, prisons, or private houses variously altered; irregular; not unfrequently, in part at least, of wood, partaking the character of huts; very defective in the cubic space allotted each inmate, and in drainage, cleanliness, and sanitary arrangements; almost invariably deficient in space for outdoor occupation and recreation, in workshops, in means of employment and amusement, and in provision for religious services; in a large proportion having no competent staff of attendants, and destitute of proper medical superintendence, being served only by nonresident medical men engaged in hospital and private practice, who visit occasionally; and, lastly, generally under no satisfactory inspection and control.

The natural consequences of such grave and numerous defects were manifested in a high rate of mortality, in the accumulation of chronic insanity, in the wide use of mechanical coercion, by manacles, strait-waistcoats, and even by chains, and in frequent recourse to seclusion, in short (to use the words of the reporters), "in the substitution of a system of imprisonment for one of cure." It is, however, only fair to state that in the American and Australian colonies the provision for the insane was on the whole more satisfactory than in the other colonial possessions.

Since 1864, and, perhaps, in part owing to the expo-

sure of their shortcomings in the returns quoted, several
of the Colonial Governments have taken steps to improve
the condition of their lunatic population and of their
asylums, and to erect new structures after the best
European models. The Governments of New South
Wales, of Victoria, and of some of the provinces of the
Dominion of Canada, deserve credit for the desire manifested to secure for the insane the best accommodation
and arrangements, and for the opportunities they have
afforded their medical officers to make themselves
acquainted with the principal institutions of Europe,
with their construction and organization, and with the
modes of treatment pursued in them.

It is in the smaller colonies generally that the condition of the insane was found most deplorable at the
date of the inquiry in 1863, and it is in these also that
the fewest attempts have yet been made at reform.
Some further action on the part of the Home Government is needed to remedy a state of things incompatible
with the requirements of humanity, and at variance with
the accepted principles of management and treatment.

WEST INDIAN COLONIES.—These are among the
oldest British colonies, and have had the longer opportunity to develop and perfect their philanthropic institutions. The opportunity, however, has been sadly
neglected, and the wretchedness and unfitness of their
receptacles for lunatics, as shown by the published
returns in 1863, were scarcely equalled in any other
colony. In the absence of later information respecting

most of them, the account then rendered must be referred to for the information following, although it is to be hoped that attention having at that period been called to their sad defects, some attempts, at least, have been made to remove them. " In the character of their buildings, and in all sanitary arrangements (so says the report), these institutions are for the most part signally defective. The buildings are in many cases old barracks, prisons, or private houses, in no way adapted for their present purpose, and wanting in every requisite for the economy of labour, or the first conditions of health. In only three out of the whole number of twenty-seven from which answers have been received, is there any tolerable provision for sewerage, drainage, and latrines. . . . Space and ventilation are equally disregarded." Here, in buildings under the tropics, there are six places where less than 500 cubic feet of space per head was allowed. " The asylum of *Dominica* gives 300 in single cells; the Vieuxfort hospital in *St. Lucia* 281 in associated wards; and the majority of the rest range from 500 to 800, and this often with the most imperfect ventilation. . . . The effects are manifest in the prevalence and destructiveness of gangrene, dysentery, and skin and bowel complaints generally."

" The asylums are crowded with mere idiots, who take nothing but harm from confinement and association with the insane. In the majority of instances there is no resident medical officer," and the proportion of nurses to inmates is insufficient. " The asylums are generally without provision for religious services, and uniformly without proper means for the amusement and employment of the insane. Curative treatment of insanity is, indeed, not yet in its infancy in the West Indian Colonies. It is, however, satisfactory to find that the idea of excessive restraint is generally repudiated even in them." There is no adequate inspection of the asylums, and the governing bodies or committees are highly objectionable in their constitution, and worse than useless in the performance of their functions.

Jamaica.—The asylum of this island was a section of the general hospital originally, and in the most wretched condition up to the time of the official report. It was, in the words of the report, "an instance of inveterate neglect;" and in the matter of suitableness for its purposes, might be "said almost to reverse every condition which ought to be observed."

The indomitable perseverance of Dr. Bowerbank, of Kingston, in exposing the wretchedness of the asylum and its inmates, and in calling for reform, was at length rewarded by the appointment of a Commission of Inquiry, and by the completion of the new asylum, projected and commenced indeed twenty years previously. Many will be familiar with the plans for the Jamaica Asylum appended to Dr. Conolly's work on the Construction of Asylums. This plan was adopted by the colonial authorities, and a commencement of an asylum, built according to it, was made; but it was soon found that the cost would very far exceed what was estimated, and that the design was unsuited to the climate and the wants of the population. The consequence

was, operations were suspended, and the partly-erected
structure lapsed into neglect and almost into ruin until
1860, when steps were taken to recommence building
an asylum. The work done up to that time was pronounced unsuitable for the object intended, and in the
end the plan was remodelled. Subsequently, under the
advice of Dr. Allen, who went out from England to
undertake the superintendence, considerable additions
have been made, and the condition of the institution is
now pronounced on the whole very satisfactory. The
average population is 1472. Mechanical restraint is
not employed, and seclusion kept within moderate
limits. Employment in the gardens, in some shops,
and about the wards, is found for the inmates, and
various means of amusement and religious services are
provided.

British Honduras.—The asylum buildings in 1863
were pronounced unsatisfactory, and the necessity of a
new structure recognized. In *Turks Islands* no asylum
existed.

British Guiana.—There is an asylum at Georgetown,
Demerara. In 1863 "no condemnation could be too
strong for the present structure; a collection of confined cells wholly unsuited for a tropical climate, almost
without means of ventilation. . . . No records of restraint are mentioned. There are absolutely no provisions for employment or amusement, and for exercise
nothing but some small covered yards. There are no
religious services. Some land which might be planted
or cultivated is suffered to be unused. Nor is this state

of things to be wondered at where there are no inspections by superior authorities, and no information is required by or furnished to the Governor." The frame of a new building was reported to be completed. This statement intimates what, in the case of many similar institutions, is distinctly stated, that the proposed new structure is to be of wood, a material highly objectionable for a public establishment like an asylum. The reporter appends the observation that "a new building will avail little if it is to inherit the bad management and the want of supervision of the old." The most recent information states that the present building is ill-adapted for an asylum in a tropical climate. It is raised 10 feet from the ground on stone pillars, and accommodates 57 patients. Mechanical restraint, the strait-waistcoat, and solitary confinement, are used occasionally. No employment and no amusements provided. There is one medical officer (non-resident), and two attendants of each sex. A fine specimen of an asylum!

Barbadoes.—The asylum was reported to be overcrowded, without day-rooms or lavatories, with only one bath-room, and very imperfectly ventilated, some rooms being even without windows. No sewerage, but cesspools annually cleared and surface drainage. Employment found for only 10 out of 58 inmates. Restraint by manacles and by seclusion very frequent. No religious services and no visits of inspection.

More recent returns indicate reforms. The asylum is about a mile and a half from the town, and is surrounded by some six acres of land. It contains 66 patients, under the care of a medical superintendent, with five male and five female attendants. Outdoor employment for the men, and exercise in airing-courts, with amusement in the shape of cards, bagatelle, and the magic lantern, are provided. Slight mechanical restraint and solitary confinement are sometimes resorted to.

Trinidad was reported as having, in 1863, no asylums, the insane being found in the hospitals and gaols. Since that period an asylum has been built about a mile and a half from Fort-of-Spain, and 150 feet above the sea level. It accommodates 42 patients. No mechanical restraint is allowed, but seclusion is resorted to at times for one to two hours. The male patients are employed in gardening, if they like it, and needlework is found for the females. The amusements comprise singing, dancing, and the lighter forms of gymnastics. There is also an harmonium. The asylum is under the care of a medical superintendent, with four male and two female attendants.

St. Vincent, Nevis, and Tobago possessed no asylum.

Grenada had a very small asylum, governed by the Board of Guardians of the poor, and not satisfactory. "There is no provision for sewerage or drainage, or, apparently, for latrines, for hot-baths, or for employment, unless in menial services. The doctor is non-resident, and visits only once in forty-eight hours; the immediate care of the lunatics being vested in a keeper and a matron at 75*l*. 12*s*. per annum, seemingly divided between the two. There are no regular reports, and visitation is rare."

St. Lucia.—The asylum is at Castries, and " it would be difficult to find any institution more defective in almost every requisite than this." The surgeon was non-resident, and visited weekly. Fortunately it contained only seven inmates generally at a time, death keeping down accumulation, for " whilst the annual admissions are stated to average only two in the last five years, there have been eight deaths as against six discharges." No occupation, no enclosures, or baths, or lavatories, or latrines, or drainage, or religious instruction, or amusements; conditions that had had their concomitants in " strait-waistcoats, manacles, and (what has no parallel in any other colony) even chains," and no record kept of such restraints. Such a den existed in a British colony in 1863.

Antigua had an asylum affording room for 48 patients. " Twenty-two of these are allowed less than 640 cubic feet per head. Strait-waistcoats, straps, manacles, and confinement are the means of restraint, and are used at the discretion of the superintendent (non-medical), who reports to the doctor. The doctor is non-resident, and visits regularly only twice a week. The patients appear to be employed chiefly in menial services." A more recent notice represents the asylum as being a satisfactory one, on a good site near the town of St. John, and accommodating 48 patients. It is superintended by a medical man, who has under him two male and two female attendants. Suitable occupation is provided, and exercise in courts. Several forms of mechanical restraint are, however, used.

Dominica possessed an asylum, formerly a military prison, and wholly unfit for the residence of lunatics. It was managed by the master of the Poor Asylum under a non-resident surgeon. It received only male patients, and had neither airing courts, nor provision for employment or amusement, and no sewerage or drainage, baths or latrines, and might be classed as a worthy companion to the buildings at St. Lucia.

Bahamas.—At Nassau is an asylum situated on the hill-side, and one storey high. Mechanical restraint in the form of manacles and irons for the feet, with solitary confinement, in extreme cases, occasionally resorted to. The institution contains 70 inmates, and has a medical superintendent, and one male attendant to every eight, and one female to every six patients.

Bermudas.—The asylum (wrote the reporter in 1863) is "perhaps the worst of all the cruelly ill-managed prisons for lunatics in the colonies; a striking instance of the results which follow from the want of any recognised system of management and inspection. . . . The site is bad and cold, the walls damp. The rooms are too few, overcrowded, ill-constructed, draughty in winter, ill-ventilated in summer, and so small as to give in some cases no more than 540 feet of space to each patient in single cells. There is no sewerage or drainage, and the latrines are mere pits without outlet of any kind, and are extremely offensive." Baths and lavatories so defective, that it may be said there are no provisions for cleanliness. No land cultivated by patients; no means for employment or exercise. The medical man is not resident, and the entire management is vested in the head-keeper. This narration recalls that given by Pinel and Esquirol of the miserable dens found in their day at the Salpêtrière.

This brief history of asylums and of the state of the insane in the West Indies affords argument for immediate action to be taken to effect a thorough reform, to rescue this country from the opprobrium of allowing a condition of things to prevail in such important colonies, discreditable to civilisation and humanity. It is clear that many of the defective and wretched arrangements are referable to the multiplication of very small institutions, to the smallness of many of the island colonies, to the deficiency of means to establish and maintain public benevolent institutions, and to the paucity of intelligent population penetrated by a due recognition of the wants of the insane, and conversant with the requirements and management of asylums. ˙Add to these causes, the want of a central controlling and supervising body—of a Commission or Board of Inspectors.

The appointment of a Commission of Inquiry for the whole of the West Indian Colonies is the first requisite ; and on the appearance of its Report, steps should be taken to adopt its recommendations, and to appoint a small permanent Commission, empowered to carry on a periodical inspection and to enforce the regulations adopted for the due care and treatment of the insane throughout the several islands. In connexion with this measure would follow the creation of several principal asylums, and the abolition of most of the small, wretched receptacles for the insane now in existence.

DOMINION OF CANADA.—In the province of Ontario (Upper Canada) are five asylums, and in that of Quebec (Lower Canada) are two. Nova Scotia, Newfoundland, New Brunswick, and Prince Edward Island, each possesses one asylum. The records of these asylums are much more satisfactory than those of the West Indian Islands, although in some of them very serious defects obtain, particularly in structural fitness.

Toronto has the oldest institution for the insane in Canada. The first building set apart for the lunatics of Upper Canada was the old gaol, situated in the centre of the town of Toronto. This was in 1841. In 1845 a special building was commenced, and in 1850 211 patients were removed to it from the previous temporary receptacles. In 1856 this new asylum was found too small, and a branch or annexe was opened in connexion with it in a building newly erected as a college in the University Park, and about two miles distant from the principal institution. It has since been carried on under the same superintendence and management, and is known as the " University Branch Asylum." On the completion of two new wings in course of erection at the parent establishment, this annexe will be given up. As an abode for the insane, its unfitness has all along been recognised.

The Toronto Asylum, when completed, will accommodate 600 patients. Dr. de Wolf (*Journal of Mental Science*, Jan. 1869, p. 466) reports it as built with a view to proper classification and furnished with all needful appliances, and heated in winter by hot water. The government despatch, however, of 1863, referred to the Toronto Asylum as not so entirely satisfactory, but as defective in its arrangements for ventilation and in the amount of land available for the purposes of recreation and employment. Two detached infirmaries (hospitals so called) have recently been erected in the grounds.

Until the British North America Act came into force in July, 1867, and since 1859, all the asylums and prisons of the two provinces were placed more or less under the control of a general board of "Inspectors of Asylums, Prisons, &c.," five in number, who inspected them and made special reports when necessary, and published also an annual return of their proceedings. Since the act above named became law, all those public institutions have been transferred to the control of the local legislatures of Ontario and Quebec, with the exception of two, the Provincial Penitentiary and the Criminal Asylum of Rockwood, which are under the exclusive jurisdiction of the Legislature of Canada, and continue to be visited and reported on by the Board of Inspectors. These official Reports have hitherto presented a large mass of details respecting the state of the several asylums and of their inmates, and of the views and projects of the medical superintendents.

In his Reports of the Toronto Asylum, Dr. Workman, the well-known zealous superintendent, has strongly urged the foundation of secondary institutions for the chronic insane, whom he proposes to transfer to them from the primary or curative establishment; and has replied to the objections generally advanced against such a scheme. Dr. Workman diligently carries out the accepted principles of moral treatment, finding outdoor work and indoor employment and amusements for his patients; but he does not accept the system of non-restraint in its entirety, believing that mechanical coercion is at times salutary. The land attached to the Toronto Asylum is about 50 acres.

Malden Asylum, originally instituted as a branch of the Toronto Asylum, and for some years placed under the same superintendence. It was a receptacle for chronic cases, but is now constituted a distinct asylum for seven counties, and has its own resident medical superintendent, Dr. Fisher. It is beautifully placed on the shore of the Detroit river, but having been originally designed for a military barrack, it has no pretensions to fitness as an asylum. Moreover, it is far too small for the population it is destined to serve, and is consequently much overcrowded. It possesses 72 acres of land, including garden space amounting to four acres. Dr. Fisher advocates its abandonment—except as a residence for incurables—and the erection of a new building near the neighbouring town of London. At the close of 1866 he reported 235 patients as remaining under treatment; 23 had been admitted in the course of the year.

Orillia Asylum, originally built for an hotel, was appropriated about eight years since, as an annexe of the Toronto Asylum, to receive chronic cases. It, however, now admits a few recent cases, and has a resident medical superintendent, Dr. Ardagh. Of the 176 admissions, to December 31st, 1866, 150 were transfers from the Toronto Asylum. During 1866, 10 admissions took place, and the population amounted to 121. It is a brick building, pleasantly situated on Lake Couchiching; but the surrounding land is very low, and not more than some 8½ acres in extent. The official despatch of 1863 commented upon the smallness of space allotted each patient — only 500 cubic feet — in the associated dormitories, on the want of land, and on the insecurity of the fences, " which necessitates either excessive confinement and restraint, or a large staff of attendants."

Rockwood Criminal Asylum. — In 1855, the insane male convicts were lodged in a portion of the Provincial Penitentiary, whilst the female convicts were placed in a temporary building at Rockwood, also in the same locality as the Penitentiary. In 1857 an act was passed to erect an asylum for all such criminal lunatics and for dangerous lunatics at large. This plan was completed, and the new building occupied at the close of 1868 by inmates of both sexes. It is built of stone, and placed on a good elevation on the shore of Lake Ontario, thereby enjoying very extensive views. During 1867, 162 patients were under treatment. The admissions were 31 in number. There is accommodation for 150 of each sex, and at the present time, happily, the demand for it, especially on the part of female convicts, is very small. "Nearly all the female lunatics," remarks Dr. Litchfield, the medical superintendent, "have from the first occupation of the temporary asylum at Rockwood been sent under warrant as 'lunatics dangerous to be at large.' At this time there is not, and for several past years there has not been, one female lunatic from the Penitentiary in the Asylum." Hence, he urges the appropriation of the unoccupied space to the reception of "pay patients of a better class," for whom suitable accommodation is much needed in Canada.

In the province of Ontario at large there is a demand for an increase of proper accommodation for the insane. The "University Branch," the Malden and the Orillia Asylums can only be accepted as temporary expedients to supply it. The rapid growth of the population of the country calls for the institution of new asylums, erected for the special object, for groups of counties, at suitable and readily accessible points.

In the province of Quebec the asylum accommodation is more scant and much inferior. Of the two asylums extant, one is a private institution at Quebec, and the other a mere makeshift near Montreal, so that in fact a proper provincial public asylum does not exist.

Beauport Asylum is a large proprietary establishment, about four miles from Quebec, opened in September, 1845. It is a stone structure, not built according to any pre-arranged asylum plan, but raised at different times to meet the demands made upon it for accommodation. It consists of two principal buildings, the one now occupied by male patients having been erected some five years since. The site is stated to be open and healthy, and there are about 100 acres of land attached to it, partly wooded, and partly cultivated.

It contained on the 1st of January, 1867, 603 patients: the admissions during the year 1866, were 153. The despatch of 1863, described the institution as at that time overcrowded, and a new structure then recently added, as defective ; but that altogether it was in a satisfactory state. In the Reports of the Inspectors, reference is made to imperfect ventilation and to the faulty system of construction, adopted in the new buildings, of placing the dormitories, like prison cells, back to back. An apology is offered by the proprietors for this structural arrangement, which, however, is both hard to understand and to appreciate. Indeed, the insight it gives into the character of the plan condemned, renders that condemnation still more deserved. Another recent addition is that of a detached house for private patients from the wealthier classes, who have, heretofore, for the most part, been sent to establishments in the United States.

A memorandum in the despatch of 1863, refers to the very frequent association of phthisis with insanity in the Canadian asylums, stating that two-thirds of the deaths in the Beauport Asylum arose from that disease ; 60 out of 145, in the Toronto ; 13 of 25 at Malden, and 18 of 105 in New Brunswick. The tables of deaths in the Beauport Asylum confirm the fact ; for of 52 deaths

T

in 1866, 22 were due to phthisis. As many as 9 were attributed to exhaustion; 3 to senile debility; 2 to gangrene; 4 to chronic diarrhœa and dysentery, whilst 2 are indefinitely assigned to "febris." These causes of death indicate a low state of health; which, so far as it does not belong to the patients at the time of admission, is suggestive of defective sanitary conditions within the establishment, such as imperfect ventilation and deficient cubic space.

The observations in the Reports, to the effect that many patients are yearly admitted who have been for months previously confined in gaols, and too often have become incurable, demonstrate the necessity of further provision for lunatics in the province of Quebec,—a necessity insisted upon in the despatch to the Colonial Office in 1863, and most reprehensibly permitted still to obtain. In that year (1863), there were 130 lunatics in gaols, and 60 others who could not obtain even that sort of accommodation.

St. John Asylum.—Not far from Montreal, is the only other receptacle in the province of Quebec for lunatics. It was formerly a court-house, which was hurriedly converted into an asylum in 1861, to receive patients who were then about to be transferred to the St. John's barracks. The buildings are partly of brick and partly frame. They stand in the centre of the village, and (says the despatch of 1863) "It is impossible to convey by words an adequate idea of the miserable condition of this asylum. Its condition is so bad that the interrogatories are said to be inapplicable."

Yet about 80 unfortunate patients are yearly "under treatment" in this place. Mr. Howard, the Medical Superintendent, says he has had to contend with this make-shift institution for six years : that " Lower Canada is in a miserable state for the want of a lunatic asylum. Beauport is more than full; St. John's in the same state."—(Report for 1866.)

New Brunswick has one asylum, established in 1848, and well placed on the banks of the St. John's River. About 75 acres are attached. Its average resident population is a little under 200, and its average yearly admissions are nearly 100. It was built for its special purpose; but the Reports a few years since alluded to structural defects, to rapid decay, to a dangerous and inefficient plan of warming, to defective kitchen and laundry arrangement; and the despatch of 1863, states it to have been without lavatories, without proper means for amusement, with no records of restraint, and no satisfactory inspection. In 1862, there was much over-crowding; but this was remedied by large additions to the building. In 1864, it was again over full and more accommodation demanded, and it is but just to Dr. Waddell, the Superintendent, to mention that in the Report for 1864, he corrected some of the statements as to defects, made in the despatch quoted. From one to two per cent. were then returned by him as under mechanical restraint or seclusion, but as he kept no record, this assertion amounts to little more than his general impression.

Newfoundland Asylum.—Situated near St. John's

town, was opened in 1847, and accommodates 120 patients.   It was sadly overcrowded in 1863; there was a
want of proper airing-courts and of means of amusement.   Dr. de Wolf says of it, that it bears an excellent
reputation, and that the returns as to its operations are
very satisfactory.   The percentage of recoveries was
stated in the Report for 1860, to be 54·7.   The number
then resident was 96; at the time the asylum was instituted (in 1847) only 17 lunatics were known to exist
in the then population of 100,000—since increased to
122,638.   It is understood that the colony is mainly
indebted to the philanthropic exertions of Miss Dix for
the possession of this asylum.

Nova Scotia.—The asylum in 1863 was reported insufficient, unfinished, crowded with helpless imbeciles,
defective in cubic capacity, and the oldest portion damp
and out of repair.   It was established in 1858; is situated on the opposite side of Halifax harbour to the
city, and commands a wide view; a new (the south)
wing was completed in 1861.   It is a brick building of good elevation, generally of three storeys;
when some additions are completed it will accommodate
300 patients.   It possesses 85 acres of land.   Its resident population was, in 1867, 167; the number has
annually augmented since its opening in 1859 with
42 patients.   The site of this satisfactory asylum was
selected by the well-known philanthropic American
lady, Miss Dix.   Dr. de Wolf, the Superintendent, reports (*op. cit.* p. 467), that in its construction all the
modern appliances have been introduced; that it is

lighted by gas made on the premises; has an unequalled water supply and excellent drainage. Very
adequate employment and amusements are provided.
From private accounts received, it appears to be one
of the best kept and managed asylums in America.
Restraint, though not abolished, is well-nigh being so.
An annual Report has been issued since its opening
in 1859.

Prince Edward's Island.—The asylum in 1863 figured
very badly in the Government Despatch and Report.
The drainage and ventilation were very bad; the cubic
capacity per patient very inadequate, and no records of
restraint were kept. It formed a section of a poor-
house. Dr. de Wolf says, "It is an alms-house with
lunatic wards (so-called) and averages about 40 patients.
The cells, for they deserve no better name, are in part
underground, with the smallest windows, no ventilation,
barely heated with stove-pipes; and altogether so re-
pulsive in their appearance as to impress the visitor
most unfavourably. This institution has no resident
physician, nor are any Reports published otherwise
than in the newspapers. The insane of the better class
are, as a matter of course, sent abroad for treatment"
(*op. cit.* p. 467).

This condition of things is disgraceful to a civilized
country.

AUSTRALIAN COLONIES and TASMANIA.—The asylums in the Australian Colonies and Tasmania have
a better reputation attaching to them. Nevertheless
their history is to a great extent a repetition of that of

the asylums in Canada and other colonies. Gaols in
the early period served as receptacles for the seclusion
of lunatics, and when those no longer sufficed for the
increasing number, then some large building or other
was transformed into an asylum, or buildings were
erected to receive the insane, but without suitable
plans, and were added to when required, without reference to a consistent general design, and rather to
suit temporary convenience and pressing circumstances.
Hence it happens that the first built asylums in Australia are now felt to be ill-suited at best for their purpose; and, by the increasing demands upon their space
consequent on increasing population, are also very inadequate in size. It is gratifying to find that the
provincial Governments are alive to the necessity of
remedying defects, and that they have shown a laudable desire to raise the state of their asylums to a level
with that of the best in Europe. The Government of
New South Wales, in particular, has shown itself so
much in earnest, that it despatched a physician (Dr.
Manning) and an architect, to Europe and America, to
visit, examine, and report upon the best asylums in
existence,—as well upon their construction as their
management and modes of treatment. Dr. Manning
having completed his tour of inspection, returned to
Sydney, and published a very complete and instructive
account of his observations and of the lessons he gathered.

New South Wales possesses two public and one
private (licensed) asylums. The lunatic asylum at
Tarban Creek has now changed name, and is known as

the Hospital for the Insane, Gladesville, near Sydney.
It was, until lately, under the superintendence of Dr.
Campbell. No return was made in answer to the
queries issued from the Colonial Office in 1863, and
only the information, in a great measure kindly contributed by Dr. Manning by letter, is at hand. In
1855, it was reported that, owing to the inadequate
means placed at the disposal of the Superintendent, the
want of accommodation and appliances, and the inherent defects of the building, classification was impossible. There was also an absence of all provision for
healthy employment and recreation for the patients,
and an objection was taken to the site as being isolated
and difficult of access. This state of things induced a
Committee of Inquiry to propose the erection of an
entirely new asylum after the best model, on a different
spot. This proposition unfortunately still awaits real-
ization.

Dr. Campbell, the Superintendent, condemned the
building in 1855, as never possibly convertible into a
fitting asylum. It was originally constructed to accommodate 60 patients. At the present time it contains
660, although its proper capacity, without crowding, is
only for 300. "Every day-room, corridor, and passage
of communication (writes Dr. Manning) is full of beds;
and as the building is badly ventilated, and the conveniences, latrines, &c., are few in number and inac-
cessible at night, the rooms are offensive to a degree
which can scarcely be credited. With all this, however, owing to the climate allowing the patients

remaining out of doors all day, their general health is excellent."

The original building has at successive periods been enlarged, but both it and the additions have the same prison-like character, although credit is taken for many improvements effected of late years. Dr. Manning's verdict is, that it is not an asylum fitted for the curative treatment of the insane. The position with regard to views of the surrounding country is good, but the windows are small, the airing courts confined, gloomy, and prison-like. "It is, besides, wanting in some of the most marked requirements of a modern hospital for the insane. It has neither amusement-hall, chapel, workshops, farm, nor proper rooms for attendants; its kitchen lacks almost all modern appliances and fittings, and will not bear comparison with even the poorest appointed of the asylums of Great Britain and the north of Europe. It is extremely difficult of access, so that the cost of victualling and stores is much increased," the visits of friends to the inmates is difficult, and opportunity cannot be had of taking patients to visit the minor amusements of Sydney, or any other large town. Further, "the great essential for the proper working of an asylum—land for cultivation—is wanting, and cannot in all probability be acquired;" and, lastly, the feeding, clothing, and means of amusement are very defective. On the other hand, the buildings are strongly constructed and in good repair.

It is very gratifying to learn that the non-restraint system of treatment was fully carried out in this insti-

tution under the management of Dr. Campbell, to
whom the credit belongs of being the first to apply that
system in a large inconvenient colonial asylum containing from 500 to 600 patients. In 1848 he was entrusted
with the superintendence, and called upon to reform the
previously existing abuses, and since that date no coercion
has been practised. Seclusion, moreover, is resorted to
only on rare occasions, as when "any internal or external cause of excitement urges a patient into an
unusual state of aggressive exaltation, or where great
activity of the suicidal propensity exists, and it is only
continued until the paroxysm in either case subsides.
Padded rooms are generally used in the instance of
suicidal patients," but the usual sleeping rooms are the
most suitable in the case of others. No interference
with the liberty of the inmates is allowed except by the
express direction of the superintendent or his deputy.
" Indeed, the very word restraint is unknown in the
asylum."

To Dr. Campbell, particular credit, writes Dr. Manning, is due for having brought the institution under
such discipline, inasmuch as the asylum has always
been sadly overcrowded, and has had above the average
proportion of violent patients (owing to the fact that
all the acute cases are sent here, and there is still a
large leaven of the old convict element).

Parramatta Asylum.—The notice of this institution
in respect to its structural fitness is not more favourable. It is spoken of as a factory and prison-like building, of gloomy appearance, and as utterly and completely

unfit for the purposes of an asylum. "In this condemnation are included the convict factory, now occupied by the women, the various buildings occupied by the insane non-criminal men, and the small prison, which has been somewhat recently erected to serve as an asylum for criminal lunatics. In such buildings the proper care and treatment of the insane is simply impossible. It needs no special knowledge on this subject to see how completely unfitted the old factory, with its gloomy, ill-ventilated cells, with their iron-barred doors, is, as a residence for those mentally afflicted. . . . . The new building for criminals seems to have been built solely with a view to the safe keeping of the inmates—a prison within an asylum—a prison and nothing more—in which treatment, in its full sense, is impossible. . . . . No amount of money or skill can avail to render Parramatta Asylum a fit residence for the insane, and its early abandonment is unhesitatingly advised."

This establishment recently contained 510 patients. Of these 51 were criminal lunatics; the remainder being chronic or incurable. No restraint is used except among the criminals, some two or three of whom are restrained by hand-cuffs and leg-irons. Some such are, as Dr. Manning expresses it, individuals who are more bad than mad, and are sometimes sent to the establishment with too much precipitancy.

Cook's River Asylum.—Licensed house,—receives 30 lunatics, of whom 25 are maintained at the public expense. Dr. Manning reports it as in every respect excellently conducted. It is also under strict regulations and frequently visited.

In the three establishments just described, 1200 lunatics are disposed of; but besides these many others are scattered through the colony, in various public buildings, including gaols as well as in private houses; and it is on all hands admitted, that additional asylums are greatly needed. It is satisfactory also to find that no attempt is to be made at establishing gigantic central institutions, but that the proposal is to construct several moderate asylums placed within convenient access of principal towns. As yet the political and financial condition of the colony has been a bar to the carrying out of this well-considered scheme.

Victoria.—*Yarra-Bend Asylum,* near Melbourne, was opened in 1848. The portion first used was built of stone, but at several successive periods additions were made of a less substantial character, of wood, some of them partaking rather of the character of sheds than of proper abodes for patients. These additions were, moreover, planned upon no general system, and the result was an irregularly and widely-dispersed collection of buildings, difficult of management and effective supervision.

The situation on one of the bends of the Yarra is good. The main building consisted of a centre, with a wing on either side. Behind each wing were two enclosed "yards," one for harmless, the other for dangerous patients; and, as if to further enhance the impression of their wild-beast character, there was, in

1853, " an open fence extending across the upper part
(of the yards), separating the attendants and visitors
from the lunatics, and allowing of easy supervision."
At the same date, likewise, the kitchen, laundry, and
cook's apartment consisted of " an old aboriginal hut,
ruinous, blackened, and inconvenient."

Patients of all classes and conditions were brought
together in this ill-arranged establishment, which yearly
became more unfit and more unmanageable, and encum-
bered with incurables.   Some seven or eight years since
its condition ˙arrested public attention, and, after an
inquiry into its whole management, it was resolved to
obtain the services of a medical superintendent trained
in an English asylum, and those of Dr. Paley were
secured.   Under the supervision of this gentleman a
thorough reform was carried out, and numerous structural improvements made.   A new building has been
projected.   Dr. Paley is now appointed Inspector of
Asylums in the colony, and has issued a Report for
1868.   From the statistical tables in this document, the
rapid development of the Yarra-Bend Asylum becomes
manifest.   It opened in October, 1848, and admitted
25 patients; in 1864, its annual admissions reached
their maximum, 350; in 1868, they were 230.   In 1866
and in 1867, the average numbers resident amounted to
1001; in 1868, they had fallen to 886.

This diminution in the population of Yarra-Bend
may be attributed to the opening of other asylums in
the colony.   In fact, during 1868, 285 were transferred
to such other institutions.   The official Report contains

memorandums of the following additional lunatic establishments:—

Carlton, Receiving-house for the Insane, admitted
113 patients during 1868, of whom 53 per cent. were
discharged recovered and relieved. " The establishment was generally in a creditable state, and, considering the nature and character of the buildings, it may
be said to answer the purpose of a receiving-house in a
satisfactory manner."

Ararat, Hospital for the Insane, was opened in October, 1867. " On the 1st of January, 1868, there were
under care 102 patients; and on the 31st of December
in the same year, the total number of inmates was 270.
" The Reports as to the condition and management of
the asylum have been satisfactory. Here, as at Beechworth, the incompleteness of the arrangements in respect
of outdoor offices and appliances, workshops, &c., has
occasioned numerous minor difficulties in the working
of the institution."

Beechworth, Hospital for the Insane, opened also in
October, 1867. " On the 1st of January, 1868, there
were 71 patients under care, and on the 31st of December, 1868, the number had increased to 295." The
management of this institution is reported as creditable
to its officers. The out-offices, airing-grounds, shops,
&c., are still incomplete.

Cremorne, Licensed Asylum, opened in October, 1867.
On the 1st of January, 1868, it had 78 residents, but
in the course of this year, 74 government patients were
transferred to Yarra-Bend, and on the 31st of December

there were left in it only eight private patients. On
every occasion when visited its condition and management were favourably reported.

Western Australia has an asylum at Fremantle.
No special information is in hand respecting it, except
the few observations on its condition contained in the
official Report of 1863. Together with the general
hospital, it is there represented to be a portion of the
convict establishment, and to be devoid of proper sewerage and drainage, and of baths and lavatories. It had
also no resident medical officer, and was almost destitute of land or of other means for the employment of
the insane. Its population was returned at 42. Its
site is low and swampy.

South Australia.—A new asylum is now in course of
construction at Adelaide.

As happens in the Canadian asylums, phthisis is a
prevailing cause of death in the lunatic hospitals of
Australia. General paresis, however, is apparently
more common in the latter colony.

TASMANIA.—" The public hospital and asylum (wrote
the reporter in 1863) are apparently faultless in every
respect, except that in the asylum three wards are very
deficient in space." It had a resident medical officer,
and its average population was returned at 264. No
mechanical restraint had for some time been resorted to.

NEW ZEALAND.—The following is an extract of
a letter from Sir George Grey, Bart., K.C.B., late
Governor of the Cape of Good Hope and New Zealand,
in reply to a written request for information concerning

the institutions for the treatment of the insane in those colonies. The information regarding New Zealand is particularly satisfactory.

May 13*th*, 1869.—" The lunatics at the Cape of Good Hope are all placed in an asylum on Robbin Island, in Table Bay. Ample Reports are yearly furnished the Colonial Government regarding the state and management of this asylum. These Reports are generally published and laid before the Cape Parliament.

" In the case of New Zealand there is more difficulty in getting information. That colony is divided into nine provinces, each of which takes care of its own lunatics, and has its own asylum. Each of these asylums is supported and managed by the provincial Government of the province in which it is situated, and the general Government of the islands exercises little or no control over them. The size and convenience of the asylums, and the amount expended on the care of the lunatics, depend therefore upon the wealth of the province and the amount of its resources.

".The province of *Auckland* has lately built a large lunatic asylum, possessing every convenience, and situated about four miles from the capital town. I have not visited it since its completion ; but from the attention bestowed on the subject, and the large sum expended in its erection, I have no doubt no expense or attention is spared in the care of the lunatics.

" The *Wellington* Asylum is small, but so, comparatively speaking, is the European population of the province. It is situated in the country, about three miles

from the capital town, and in a very healthy locality.
The superintendent or chief medical officer of the province of Wellington is a medical man of known ability,
and the asylum there is necessarily controlled by him
and under his direction; and although I have never
visited it, and therefore cannot speak from personal
knowledge, I presume with the advantages it possesses
it must be thoroughly well conducted.

"The province of *Canterbury* has a roomy and very
convenient lunatic asylum in the immediate vicinity of
Christchurch, the capital town. Taking an interest in
this asylum, I can speak of it from personal knowledge.
A large number of persons in Christchurch also take a
great interest in it, and it is most admirably conducted.
The patients are treated with great care and kindness.
The number of patients not being very large, great
consideration can be shown to each of them. In some
respects they rather seem members of a family than
patients in an asylum.

"The province of *Otago* has also a very convenient
lunatic asylum close to the capital town, Dunedin. I
am well acquainted with that asylum also. It is conducted with the greatest care, and the patients are
treated with an extraordinary degree of kindness. The
number of patients is not large, and many of the ablest
and most influential people in Dunedin take a deep
interest in their welfare. I should think, therefore,
that their life is as happy as it can be. It certainly
appears to be so. I do not know that anything has
ever touched me or pleased me more than visiting the

lunatic asylums in Christchurch and Dunedin, with the able and benevolent people who were interested in them. I have never seen human nature under a better or more attractive aspect than in the care of these people for the lunatics.

"I am not personally acquainted with the asylums in the other provinces, but I have no doubt they follow as closely as they can the models afforded them in the provinces of which I have spoken. The natives, who live in small agricultural communities scattered throughout a great extent of country, have generally a strong objection to allowing their lunatics to be confined. They leave them at large, and bestow such care on them as they can. When they are very violent, they bind them for a time with pieces of flax. It is worthy of remark that whilst they thus leave their lunatics at large, they sometimes in bad cases of leprosy confine the lepers within fences."

Besides the information conveyed in this interesting letter from Sir George Grey, other is contained in official Colonial Reports. Action has, of late years, been much paralysed by war in respect of many internal improvements, and among others making due provision for the insane; but the scheme has been accepted by the several provinces to erect a large general asylum, and the site fixed upon for it was near Nelson. The only objection to the site is that the country is liable to earthquakes, and that, in consequence, the asylum cannot be built solidly of stone or brick. The policy

U

of attempting to provide for the lunatics of several widely-extended provinces in a large central institution is very doubtful. Such an institution must ere long grow to an unwieldy size; the supervision of each province over its affairs and its inmates must be materially sacrificed, and, what is more, its distance from the greater part of the population it serves, and the difficulties of access to it, must lessen its usefulness in all ways.

Auckland Asylum, according to official returns, contained 39 patients in 1859, and 40 in 1861. The house was overcrowded. Employment was afforded to a portion only of the inmates; amusements—games, books, and music—were provided. Restraint was not used, and seclusion but little resorted to. It was under the care of Dr. McGauran, the Provincial Surgeon, who however was not resident.

Otago.—The asylum at Dunedin is a temporory structure, erected in 1863 for 30 patients, and overcrowded. Previously to its construction, lunatics were kept in the general hospital, or confined in the gaol.

Wellington.—The provincial asylum is at Karori. It consists of a long wooden building, containing 13 bedrooms, besides two sitting-rooms, kitchen, and servants' rooms. A small detached portion contains a padded and three single rooms for dirty cases. It has five acres of land attached. The medical man is non-resident, and visits only twice a week. Occupation in the garden is encouraged. Restraint is at times employed. Its population has reached 20 in number, but is usually about 12. No provision is made for religious services.

Nelson has no properly constituted asylum. Some buildings at Taranaki were temporarily used, chiefly for female patients. Other lunatics were confined in gaols, and two or three demented patients were detained in the general hospital.

Canterbury.—The provincial asylum is at Sunnyside. It is a wooden structure, and was opened in 1863. Lunatics were previously kept in Lyttleton gaol, and had augmented to 17 in number prior to the establishment of the asylum. In the first six months after its opening, 29 patients were added. In 1867 the number had increased to 75; a range of new buildings was added, and the previously very limited area of land around it was increased. The kitchen is complained of as being too small, and there are no religious services provided. A library is formed, various games are provided, and there is an asylum band. The Report is made by the steward, who uses restraint occasionally, but gives preference to seclusion in the padded room in troublesome cases. The medical officer is non-resident.

The very brief returns made to the Colonial Office are insufficient for arriving at an accurate conception of the precise condition of these New Zealand asylums and of their inmates. It is clear from Sir George Grey's remarks that the asylums exhibit an air of great comfort and the aspect of kind treatment towards the patients ; but, to the professional mind, the memoranda furnished are suggestive of very imperfectly arranged asylums and buildings, useful only as temporary receptacles for lunatics. Exception might be taken to their construction in wood, chiefly on account of the greater danger of fire, but this circumstance of structure may be deemed almost necessary in those districts subject to earthquakes. There seems, moreover, small attention given to employment, and in some of the asylums there is an insufficiency of land. The employment of mechanical coercion is more common than it should be; this and other defects in administration may be assigned to the absence of resident medical officers—an evil in existence in each of the asylums noticed.

AFRICAN COLONIES.—*Cape of Good Hope.*—The Cape Asylum on Robbin Island figures in the Report of 1863. It returned a population of 156 patients under the superintendence of a resident medical officer. " It suffers," wrote the reporter, " both from want of connection with any central medical authorities who might exercise supervision and suggest improvements, and from an anomalous subordination to the Somerset (general) Hospital. The lunatics are admitted to the hospital, and then handed over to the asylum, an arrangement which frequently results in the loss or detention of the certificates and other preliminary documents relating to the proofs, causes, and previous nature of the disease." The cubic space per patient was only 500 feet. " There is reason to believe that excessive and arbitrary use of seclusion and restraint prevails, . . . and the asylum is in a very bad state. . . . The sewerage, drainage, latrines, water-supply, lavatories, and baths have been, and indeed even at the present time still appear to be, bad and defective in the extreme. There is no system of subordination among the attendants, who seem to have been left to perform their duties in their own way, without check or supervision. The patients are employed in menial services, and frequently subjected to restraint on frivolous grounds."

It is to be hoped that these grave defects have ere this been remedied, and a proper asylum under due superintendence provided. There must also be need of asylum accommodation for the districts, as for instance Graham's-town and Port Elizabeth, at long distances from Table Bay.

Natal.—The Grey's Hospital was a compound establishment of lunatic asylum and poor-house. Its total population in 1863 was 113. It was devoid of artificial sewerage and drainage, and consisted of wards with rooms on either side a central passage or corridor. It had a resident medical officer.

Sierra Leone was returned in 1863 as having an asylum very defective in sanitary arrangements, with 68 inmates, five attendants, and a non-resident medical officer. The general verdict respecting this, the Robbin Island, and St. Helena Asylums, is that they are badly constructed and badly managed.

St. Helena.—The asylum is a parochial institution, and the parish authorities contract with a private person for the care of the insane. It has no regular medical attendant; the parish doctor visiting only when summoned by the keeper. No employment provided, and no registers or records kept. In 1863 the average number under treatment was returned as only eight.

Gambia and the Gold Coast have no asylums.

Mauritius.—The asylum in 1863 was not well placed, and small; but, except that it was deficient in means for occupation and amusement, dependent on its limited site, was not otherwise open to much objection. A new building on another site of adequate space was projected. Its population was returned as 130. From the latest account obtainable it appears to be situated about two miles from Port Louis, and not to have been constructed for its particular object. This is equivalent to saying that the poor lunatics are not comfortably lodged, and cannot be properly treated. Mechanical restraint is stated not to be employed, but it is to be feared that the internal condition of the asylum is not very satisfactory.

MEDITERRANEAN STATIONS.—*Gibraltar* had a small receptacle for lunatics in 1863, which received four or five cases yearly. It formed a part of the gaol premises, and was without land, and seemed " to be very badly managed by a superintendent and his wife with 80*l.* per annum, and a male assistant keeper with only 25*l.*, without allowances." No employment and no provision for exercise, except in walking the yards. Records, visits, and reports were all very insufficient.

Malta.—The lunatics of this island were formerly confined in an old mansion, once the residence of a knight named Frascati, situated within the city of Valetta; but since 1856 a new asylum has been erected in the country, about four miles from the capital. It is a well-built structure of stone, and is under the superintendence of a resident medical officer. It is stated to be a model of cleanliness and order, and the entire management is reported by Dr. Sutherland and other good judges to be admirable, under the humane and judicious direction of the Hon. J. V. Inglott, the Comptroller of Charitable Institutions in Malta, to whom is due the merit of making the asylum what it is. There are 43 patients—21 males and 22 females. The treatment is most humane. Restraint is rarely used ; occupation and amusements and all other means for the comfort and restoration of the inmates are promoted. Baths are in daily use, and the "Turkish bath" is considered a most powerful remedial agent in that climate. The number of cures is returned at from 43 to 46 per cent. Registers and cases recording the history of each case are kept.

Ceylon—has an asylum specially built for its purpose, and reported as well adapted. It was intended to accommodate 300 patients, but at present contains only 193, viz., 133 males and 60 females. The treatment is conducted on the non-restraint system. Seclusion is resorted to only when the patient is excited and dangerous to others or to himself, and then only by the authority of the resident medical superintendent. It is moreover always registered in a book kept for the purpose. The male patients are employed in outdoor, and the female in indoor occupations. Amusements, such as bagatelle, draughts, backgammon, are provided, and also books.

The asylum is visited by the Colonial Inspector-General
of Hospitals. The account of this asylum is in all respects
satisfactory, and highly creditable to the management
of the medical superintendent and to the authorities
under whose care it is placed.

Of few other colonial asylums in other parts of the
world is information at hand or readily attainable.

APPENDIX C.

NOTE ON THE STATE OF THE INSANE IN INDIA.

A SERIES of queries regarding the treatment of the insane throughout our dominions in India was circulated about two years ago, by order of the Right Honourable Sir Stafford Northcote, Secretary of State for India in Council. The result of this inquiry discloses one circumstance, which it has been very gratifying to learn, namely, that *non-restraint* is the principle of treatment in all the asylums of India. This general adoption of the non-restraint system, and the efforts which have been made to promote the industrial occupation of the patients, and to secure for them the means of exercise in the open air and suitable amusements, are no doubt due to the energy of our army medical officers, under whose superintendence the asylums of India are placed, and who furnish annually to the Government interesting and valuable Reports as to the state of each asylum.

Much in the way of improvement and progress has certainly been effected, but it is beyond question that much still remains to be done, in order to render the provisions for the insane in India as satisfactory as they should be, and to enable the medical officers to give practical effect to the enlightened views which they often express in their reports.

In order to promote this, a summary of the information, which the inquiry referred to yielded, will be submitted to the Secretary of State for India as soon as it can be prepared.

LONDON: PRINTED BY W. CLOWES AND SONS, DUKE STREET, STAMFORD STREET,
AND CHARING CROSS.